LABOR PAINS
MODERN MIDWIVES
AND HOME BIRTH

Deborah A. Sullivan
and Rose Weitz

Yale University Press
New Haven and London

Designed by Nancy Ovedovitz and set in Baskerville type by The Composing Room of Michigan, Inc. Printed in the United States of America by Braun-Brumfield, Inc., Ann Arbor, Michigan.

Library of Congress Cataloging-in-Publication Data

Sullivan, Deborah A., 1947–
  Labor pains.
  Includes bibliographies and index.
  1. Midwives—United States.   2. Midwives—United States—History.   3. Midwives—Social aspects.
I. Weitz, Rose, 1952– . II. Title.
[DNLM: 1. Midwifery—trends. WQ 160 S949L]
RG960.S85 1988   618.2′0233   87-23004
ISBN 0-300-04093-8 (alk. paper)

The paper in this book meets the guidelines for permanence and durability of the Committee on Production Guidelines for Book Longevity of the Council on Library Resources.

10   9   8   7   6   5   4   3   2   1

CONTENTS

PREFACE

This book explores the reemergence of midwifery and home birth. It began eight years ago, when the Arizona Bureau of Maternal and Child Health asked one of us to analyze a statewide survey of recent mothers concerning satisfaction with maternity care. The bureau wanted to understand why many women advocate changes in obstetrical practices and, in some cases, give birth at home. It seemed an ideal short-term project for Deborah, who was about to start a maternity leave. She had no idea that this project would lead to six years of studying midwives and home birth.

At the time, we were unaware of the increase in lay midwives practicing legally and illegally in the United States. We assumed, like most Americans, that midwives practiced only in impoverished communities and foreign countries. The survey of recent mothers changed that stereotype. Arizona had recently reactivated a system for licensing lay midwives who conduct home birth. The survey results suggested that at least some American women decide to use midwives for ideological rather than economic reasons. Although only a small fraction of the respondents had used licensed midwives, those few described their experiences in glowing terms. They extolled the midwives for allowing couples to make their own decisions, rather than forcing them to accept medical practices the couples considered dangerous. These respondents further claimed that home birth had spared them the anxieties and indignities of hospital birth and had allowed them to benefit from the presence of friends and family. Their remarks sounded wonderful to Deborah, who had had to struggle during two hospital births to avoid procedures that seemed unnecessarily invasive.

Aware of the potential dangers of childbirth, however, Deborah continued to question the wisdom of licensing lay midwives. Consequently, when the Bureau of Maternal and Child Health asked her to compile statistics on the health outcomes of midwife-attended home births, she accepted readily. These statistics (included in chapter 6) demanded a reassessment of the assumption that midwife-attended home births entail undue risks for low risk women.

The good outcomes further sparked our interest in midwifery. At this time we began to collaborate in designing and conducting a study of licensed midwives. The resulting interviews focused on how and why women become midwives and on the labor problems they face in a health care system dominated by male physicians. Deborah subsequently conducted similar interviews with midwives in another state who worked without legal approval. These two sets of interviews provide the basis for chapters 3, 5, and 8.

The midwives we interviewed identified opposition from physicians who regard them as dangerous quacks as the major obstacle that they face. To gauge the accuracy of the midwives' reports and to gain insight into physicians' views, we conducted a mailback survey of Arizona obstetrician-gynecologists and general and family practitioners. These data, reported in chapter 7, verify the midwives' complaints and suggest some reasons for physician hostility.

Many midwives we interviewed spoke enviously of the far higher status that midwives hold in other developed societies. Sabbatical leaves from our university allowed us to investigate the position of midwives elsewhere and to look at the conditions that make cooperation between midwives and physicians possible. Rose chose Great Britain and Deborah chose Australia and New Zealand because of the historic and continuing links between these countries and the United States. Chapter 9 presents historical, interview, and survey data on the role of midwives working in homes and hospitals in these three countries.

Our cross-cultural studies intensified our belief that to present a full picture of midwives' current role we needed to consider how our health care system had developed. The final stage in writing this book consisted of historical and legal research. This research (described in chapters 1, 2, and 4) allowed us to see how physicians gained near-total control of the American health care system, how this control has translated into law, and the dangers this medical monopoly presents to consumers.

When we began our research, we thought we had chosen a small and easily manageable topic. We now recognize that the issues involved in the reemergence of midwifery and home birth are far broader. We hope that this book will provide readers with a better understanding of how health care occupations and systems develop, the consequences of medical monopoly, and the potential for true changes in health care delivery.

ACKNOWLEDGMENTS

Many individuals and institutions have provided assistance to us in researching this book. Ruth Beeman, former director of the Arizona Bureau of Maternal and Child Health, brought to our attention the maternity care reform movement and the reemergence of lay midwives. Ruth initiated the Arizona survey of satisfaction with maternity care and the system for collecting data on midwife-attended births. Her endorsement encouraged the licensed midwives to cooperate with us, and her views about midwifery undoubtedly have influenced us. Subsequent directors of Arizona's midwifery program also provided assistance. Lisa Hulette, in particular, spent considerable time rereading virtually every case report of a transferred mother or baby and checking the accuracy of the state's records on birth outcomes.

Other individuals, many of whom worked for local, national, or international maternity reform organizations, kindly responded to our requests for information on home birth and midwifery. Although we lack the space needed to list their names, we would like to state our appreciation for their cooperation. Their commitment to improving the quality of maternity care deserves recognition.

Our own institution, Arizona State University, nurtured this book's development in several ways. Deborah received faculty grant-in-aid funds to tape and transcribe interviews with midwives in the northeastern state and Rose received grant-in-aid funds for her research in Great Britain. Sabbatical support gave both of us time and money to collect cross-cultural data. Graduate research assistance from our department made our tasks considerably easier. Elizabeth McNulty and Rumiko Nakai helped with various aspects of our work.

Kathi Fairman deserves special thanks for the many extra hours she
spent on the physician survey and the graceful way she coped with
our sabbatical departures. We left her literally at the computer, holding the data, and depending on the whims of international mail for
communication with us. We are also indebted to Debbie McGee, Victoria Martinez, Lorelle Adams, and the university word processing
staff, who cheerfully and efficiently transcribed our interviews, un-
daunted by occasional foreign accents and expressions. We especially
want to thank Debbie McGee, whose excellent typing and amiable
spirit throughout endless drafts of this book made her an invaluable
asset.

The Social Science and Administration Department of Gold-
smiths' College of the University of London, the Demography Department of Australian National University, and the Sociology Department of the University of Waikato in New Zealand graciously
provided bases for us during our overseas research. The University
of Waikato also paid for the typing and reproduction of the New
Zealand questionnaires.

Our family and friends provided essential emotional support and
sounding boards for ideas throughout this project. One friend, Con-
nie Breece, additionally interviewed two midwives in the northeastern state who were not available during the research visit. Jean
Donnison deserves a special note of thanks for taking a stray Yank
into her London home for a year.

Portions of this manuscript first appeared in somewhat different
form in *Social Problems* 33(3):163–75, February 1986, and in *Sociology
of Health and Illness*, 7:36–54, March 1985. We are grateful to the
publishers for granting us permission to reprint this material.

Finally, we wish to thank the midwives who made this book possible
by opening their homes and their thoughts as well as their work for
our scrutiny. We have tried to present their views accurately but must
bear full responsibility for our conclusions regarding the past, present, and future of midwifery and home birth.

LABOR PAINS

CHAPTER 1
THE DECLINE OF
TRADITIONAL MIDWIFERY
IN AMERICA

Throughout history, women have turned to one another for both emotional support and technical assistance during childbirth. Midwives are mentioned in some of the earliest Western writings, including Genesis 35:17. A midwife was among the Mayflower settlers (Litoff, 1978:4), and midwives delivered the majority of American babies until about 1910 (Litoff, 1978:27; Donegan, 1984:302). Traditional midwives still attend from 60 to 80 percent of births in the developing world (*Population Reports*, 1980:1), and modern midwives remain the most important providers of routine maternity care in Europe (World Health Organization, 1985:14). In the United States, however, childbirth is now viewed as a potentially dangerous event that requires extensive medical monitoring and intervention. As a result, 99 percent of births in the United States in 1983 occurred in hospitals, and 98 percent of these were attended by physicians (National Center for Health Statistics, 1985:5). This chapter will describe how American childbirth practices evolved and how midwives lost their occupational territory.[1]

1. This chapter draws heavily on several excellent histories of midwifery and childbirth. Wertz and Wertz (1977) provide a comprehensive overview of American childbirth practices. Donegan (1978) describes the changing role of midwives and physicians in early America, while Litoff's (1978) analysis takes up the story in 1860. Paul Starr's *The Social Transformation of American Medicine* (1982) offers an invaluable description of the context in which changes in childbirth

CHILDBIRTH IN EARLY AMERICA

Throughout the Colonial period and until the mid-eighteenth century, childbirth in America was attended almost solely by women (Wertz and Wertz, 1977:1). Most women gave birth in their homes or their mothers' homes, attended by midwives, female friends, and female relatives. Midwives generally let nature take its course, since dependable food supplies and the lack of crowding in the New World made childbirth a relatively safe event for white women (Wertz and Wertz, 1977:1, 19). Midwives' primary tasks were to provide emotional and spiritual support and to help the new mother with domestic chores. The word *midwife*, which comes from the Anglo-Saxon for "with woman," reflects the scope of midwives' position in women's lives.

Colonial American midwives worked under an incomplete system of municipal licensure. Where licensure existed, and unlike on the European continent, it was not accompanied by training programs. As in Britain, American midwives were considered moral guardians rather than health care providers. Civil and religious authorities rarely interfered in midwives' practices unless witchcraft or other heresy was suspected (cf. Ehrenreich and English, 1973; Forbes, 1966).[2] Those few localities that licensed midwives did so based more on character than technical expertise (Donegan, 1978:90–93; Wertz and Wertz, 1977:7–8, 12). Licensing regulations required only that midwives attended all who needed their services, revealed the truth about illegitimacy and infanticide, and foreswore abortions and magic. Colonial authorities valued midwives as sources of information about these crimes. In several instances midwives were paid salaries in recognition of their role in protecting civil order (Donegan, 1978:90; Wertz and Wertz, 1977:8). Midwives also were respected because they helped communities to grow, and thus to demonstrate their apparently favored position in the eyes of God.

Prior to the late eighteenth century, physicians and their barber-

---

practices occurred, while Jean Donnison (1977) offers the reader a crucial comparison between the histories of British and American midwives.

2. For example, suspicions that midwife Margaret Jones practiced witchcraft resulted in 1648 in her achieving "the dubious distinction of becoming the first person executed in the colony of Massachusetts Bay" (Donegan, 1978:91).

surgeon predecessors almost never attended births except when midwives or family members requested their aid with desperate, pathological cases. Physicians' role was usually limited to sacrificing the life of the fetus or the mother in the hope of saving the other. In most cases, this meant destroying and removing the fetus after a difficult, prolonged labor without progress. More rarely, physicians performed cesarean sections on dead or dying women; these operations occasionally saved infants but almost invariably killed their mothers. Sometimes both mother and fetus died, owing to poor medical skills, septic conditions, and the lack of anesthesia.

Male attendance at childbirth outside of emergencies met fierce opposition initially. When Francis Rayus tried to work as a "man midwife" in Massachusetts in 1646, for example, he was fined fifty shillings for his audacity in adopting what was considered a woman's role. Licensing procedures for Colonial midwives generally included swearing an oath not to allow men into the lying-in chamber "unless necessity or great urgent cause" required it (Donegan, 1978:18).

THE EMERGENCE OF OBSTETRICS

Man-midwifery, or obstetrics as it was called after 1828, developed in this country largely in response to European influences. Although the first American medical school opened in 1765, the quality of medical education remained inferior to that in Europe for the next 150 years. As a result, some wealthier Americans sought better training abroad during the late eighteenth and early nineteenth centuries. There they encountered the French postrevolutionary emphasis on observing human physiology, the course of diseases, and the effectiveness of treatments (Starr, 1982:54). They also learned of English forceps, techniques for turning malpositioned fetuses, and the use of opium for pain relief and ergot to stimulate labor and delivery. Armed with this scientific perspective and new technologies, physicians came back with some hope for improving the outcomes of abnormal births. They also came back with a more positive regard for man-midwifery. One of these men, William Shippen, became the first physician to teach midwifery in America in 1762 (Donegan, 1978:116). He and his students became the vanguard of a movement to redefine childbirth as a pathological event requiring monitoring and intervention by medical men.

Physicians' increasing interest in obstetrics formed part of a larger struggle to establish and expand their occupational status, authority, and autonomy (Starr, 1982:30–59). Unlike elite European physicians in the eighteenth and early nineteenth centuries, most American physicians were drawn from the working class and had little prestige. Few could afford to go abroad for training. Neither the public nor the legal system granted any more respect or privileges to "regular" physicians than to barber-surgeons, apothecaries, or the many "irregular" lay healers who took up part-time medical practice in increasing numbers in the nineteenth and early twentieth centuries. Public skepticism about these practitioners was not unreasonable. Most were poorly trained entrepreneurs whose "heroic medicine"—bleeding, blistering, and purging—did more harm than good. Some found that there was more money to be made in training than practicing. By 1850 there were 42 schools at a time when France had only 3; by 1900 there were 160 (Starr, 1982:42, 112). Medical titles could be purchased or simply adopted with little or no education, and licensure, where it existed, was merely honorific. Until the mid-nineteenth century, many medical students did not witness a single birth (Wertz, 1983:15), and as late as 1911, even students at the better medical schools typically observed fewer than five labors (Williams, 1986:90).

Attempts by physicians to increase their role, authority, and status met strong resistance during the early nineteenth century (Starr, 1982:30–59). Professional authority and licensure were rejected by both the public and legislators as dangerously elitist. Jacksonian America's ideological commitment to egalitarianism and democracy encouraged faith in the ability and self-sufficiency of the common people, including their ability to treat illness. Support grew for public education and the popular press, including the publication of medical manuals for lay persons. These manuals were well-received, especially in rural areas, where few could afford to purchase health care and most families doctored themselves. Jacksonian values facilitated the development of a large and widespread Popular Health Movement in reaction to regular medicine's excesses and shortcomings (Starr, 1982:47–54). The movement included supporters of Thomsonian botanics, homeopaths, eclectics, bonesetters, abortionists, patent medicine sellers, and Indian doctors, as well as midwives.

The public's disinclination and limited ability to pay for health care, coupled with the vast oversupply of health care practitioners, placed severe economic pressures on physicians. In response, physicians attempted to expand their role in several directions: pulling teeth, embalming the dead, sitting up with the sick, and caring for livestock, as well as attending childbirth (Starr, 1982:85). Physicians considered obstetrical work particularly crucial; they believed that families who came to a physician for childbirth would stay with him for other services (Donegan, 1978:141–42; Wertz and Wertz, 1977:55). As Dr. John Quackenbush rhetorically asked his students at Albany Medical College, "Who holds the key, that opens a large practice to the general practitioner, if the accoucheur [childbirth attendant] does not?" (1855:14).

Yet resistance to man-midwives diminished slowly. This opposition rested not only on the broader hostility to medical authority that existed in the Jacksonian period but also on prevailing social norms. Physicians' traditional association with death in childbirth stoked women's fear of male practitioners. More important, however, many social commentators equated man-midwifery with sexual licentiousness and questioned the motives of physicians who chose to work with women's bodies. As one example, a book written by a Boston physician and entitled *Man-Midwifery Exposed and Corrected* warned that "the unlimited intimacy between a numerous profession and the female population silently and effectually wears away female delicacy and professional morality, and tends, probably more than any other cause in existence, to undermine the foundations of public virtue" (Gregory, 1848:18). Apocryphal stories abounded of man-midwives who seduced their patients (Donegan, 1978:167–69; Wertz and Wertz, 1977:97–98).

To placate their critics, physicians avoided physical examinations whenever possible (Donegan, 1978:155–57; Wertz and Wertz, 1977:81–93). When examinations were unavoidable, they kept their patients' bodies covered and worked in dark rooms, relying on their sense of touch rather than vision. Fear of public censure led the fledgling American Medical Association (AMA) in 1851 to oppose the use of speculums, which it felt would embarrass women by exposing their genitalia.

These compromises severely restricted physicians' ability to practice effectively in the nineteenth century. To overcome women's opposition to male practitioners and to gain their acceptance, physicians played on women's fears of childbirth, arguing that its dangers necessitated skilled medical assistance rather than an ignorant midwife's attendance (Donegan, 1978:151–52). Physicians hoped that a woman would allow "the knowledge of her danger to override this delicacy of her feelings and the modesty of her nature" (Quackenbush, 1855:7).

THE SHIFT TO PHYSICIANS BEGINS

Despite cultural resistance to male childbirth attendants, their use increased steadily throughout most of the nineteenth century. Almost all upper- and middle-class women in northern cities used physicians rather than midwives by 1820 (Donegan, 1978:141).

The shift to physicians was supported by the Protestant view of illness as a moral rather than a magical phenomenon (Starr, 1982:35; Wertz and Wertz, 1977:22–25). Rejection of magical explanations for the world in the long run allowed individuals to begin looking for laws in nature, as religion lost its stranglehold on American culture and God became viewed as a more distant force. This laid the groundwork for conceptualizing illness as a natural rather than supernatural occurrence.

The rational conception which underlies the scientific approach was readily accepted in the United States. Starr (1982:59) argues that the development of science broke popular self-confidence in one's own ability to manage health through common sense and restored a belief in the complexity of health and illness. This in turn lowered the cultural barriers against physicians' continuing claims to authority and status. Physicians embraced scientific knowledge as the basis for a campaign to convince the public that health care required more than patent medicines, botanics, spinal manipulations, colonics, and other alternative therapies. As scientific ideas gained sway, even childbirth increasingly was seen as too complex for lay persons, especially women, to understand. As a result, the Popular Health Movement weakened and the cultural authority of medicine grew.

The growth in science also bolstered physicians' position by redefining women's experience of childbirth pain. As social stratification increased during the post-Colonial era, society began to expect upper- and middle-class women to be idle, even physically weak, as evidence of their cultured delicacy and husbands' wealth. These women probably needed pain relief more than their foremothers had, since they entered the birthing chamber with muscles tensed by fear, ribcages and pelvises deformed by corsets, and their natural strength weakened by lack of exercise, too frequent pregnancies, and tuberculosis (Wertz, 1983:18). As scientific ideas replaced religious fatalism, women became able to accept pain relief, available only from physicians, without risking the accusation that they were circumventing God's will (Wertz and Wertz, 1977:110–13).

Nineteenth-century ideas about women also encouraged the use of physicians by altering the population of midwives. Victorian society considered "true" women incapable of learning technical skills and stigmatized any who tried to do so (Welter, 1966). The influential physician and medical professor Charles Meigs, for example, wrote that a woman "has a head almost too small for intellect but just big enough for love" (1848:47). In such a climate, midwives were excluded from scientific advances in obstetrics. Most midwives could not afford the new clinical tools, could find neither sellers nor training in their use, or rejected them as men's "meddlesome midwifery" (Wertz and Wertz, 1977:39). Although a handful of physicians briefly held midwifery classes for women, potential students' lack of funds and qualms about propriety kept enrollment low (Donegan, 1984: 310; Wertz and Wertz, 1977:44–46). It was no longer acceptable for affluent Victorian women to pursue vocational training. Increasingly, parturient women of means were forced to choose between men physicians from their own class and midwives from the lower class. Many selected physicians not only in hopes of reducing childbirth's dangers and pain but also because physicians' gender and higher fees made them status symbols (Wertz, 1983:12; Leavitt, 1986:39).

Ironically, despite women's hopes, medical care presented equal if not greater dangers than midwifery care (Donegan, 1978:143–47;

Leavitt, 1983:281–92; 1986:43–58). The hazards of nineteenth-century heroic medicine are evident in Wertz and Wertz's description of a Boston woman who

> had convulsions a month before her expected delivery. The doctors bled her of 8 ounces and gave her a purgative. The next day she again had convulsions, and they took 22 ounces of blood. After 90 minutes she had a headache, and the doctors took 18 more ounces of blood, gave emetics to cause vomiting, and put ice on her head and mustard plasters on her feet. Nearly four hours later she had another convulsion, and they took 12 ounces, and soon after, 6 more. By then she had lapsed into a deep coma, so the doctors doused her with cold water but could not revive her. Soon her cervix began to dilate, so the doctors gave ergot to induce labor. Shortly before delivery she convulsed again, and they applied ice and mustard plasters again. In six hours she delivered a stillborn child. After two days she regained consciousness and recovered. The doctors considered this a conservative treatment, even though they had removed two-fifths of her blood in a two-day period, for they had not artificially dilated her womb or used instruments to expedite delivery. (1977:69)

Even when mothers survived birth, permanent injuries could be caused by overaggressive surgical intervention. Some women had to withdraw permanently from social interaction because of constantly seeping, foul tears between vagina and anus or bladder, for which no cure existed before 1849. Midwives' clients also suffered such injuries, but Bogdan (1978) argues that they would have occurred less often since midwives relied primarily on passive techniques.

Surgical intervention also endangered women by inviting infection. The primary cause of maternal mortality, "childbed" or puerperal fever, plagued hospitals since physicians moved from general surgery and autopsies to gynecological examinations, and from patient to patient, without cleaning their hands, clothes, or instruments. Physician Ignaz Semmelweis proved the contagiousness of puerperal fever in 1847 after realizing that the mortality rate was three times higher among physicians' clients than among midwives' clients (Semmelweis, 1983). The latter were less at risk, not because midwives understood the cause of sepsis and the need for precaution, but because midwives did not conduct surgery or dissections, performed fewer internal examinations and surgical interventions, worked with fewer clients, and washed more often in the process of domestic chores (Bogdan, 1978). Unfortunately for their patients, most physicians did not accept Semmelweis's conclusions for another forty years.

THE CAMPAIGN AGAINST MIDWIVES

Between 1850 and 1930, physicians lobbied effectively to better their position (Starr, 1982:93–144). The AMA was organized for this purpose in 1847, although it had little power for the next several decades. Regular physicians' first success was in removing the threat from homeopaths and eclectics. Realizing that so many medical sects diminished their credibility, regulars began to eliminate the futile heroic practices that the public resisted and to accept homeopaths and eclectics into their schools, societies, and referral networks in the mid-nineteenth century. This acceptance eventually cost homeopaths and eclectics their unique identity, as they were incorporated into mainstream medicine. Coming at a time when scientific knowledge was growing and gaining respect, this consolidation helped restore the public's belief in the "legitimate complexity" of health care and the legitimacy of physician authority (Starr, 1982:140). The new faith in science provided the cultural basis for the rejection of lay practitioners. By the time the new medical sects of Christian Science, osteopathy, and chiropractic emerged in the 1890s, physicians had sufficient power to press successfully for restrictive licensing laws. Subsequent medical lobbying efforts combined with Progressive Era legislative attacks on deceptive business practices to produce modest success in excluding patent medicine sellers and other irregulars.

Physicians' position improved significantly in the wake of the 1910 Flexner Report. This scathing indictment of the lack of scientific training in medical education won public support for an AMA-administered program of medical school accreditation to go with state licensure. This tightening of standards added to the growing public respect for physicians and greatly aided their efforts to gain control of the health care field.

The final push to eliminate midwives was one part of this larger, two-pronged, campaign to improve the quality of health care and establish medical hegemony. Physicians had begun to voice their opposition to midwives during the nineteenth century but significantly escalated their attack in the early twentieth century. Midwives were particularly vulnerable at this time, even though they still conducted the majority of American births, because they were mostly uneducated poor black and immigrant women (Kobrin, 1984:318).

Physicians' crusade against midwives reflected their economic and political interests. The tremendous influx of immigrants around the turn of the century had swelled the ranks of midwives and made their existence more visible and threatening to physicians, whose status, especially in obstetrics, remained low (Litoff, 1986:27). To gain professional standing, obstetricians had to convince both the general and medical communities that obstetrical skills were necessary, scientific, and on a par with those of other physicians. To do so, they had to denigrate midwives, whose practices suggested that childbirth did not require medical skills. Joseph B. De Lee, the foremost obstetrician of the early twentieth century, recognized this when he wrote in 1915, "If an uneducated woman of the lowest classes may practice obstetrics [midwifery], is instructed by doctors, and licensed by the State, it certainly must require very little knowledge and skill—surely it cannot belong to the science and art of medicine" (1986:102). De Lee believed that "for many centuries, she [the midwife] prevented obstetrics from obtaining any standing at all among the sciences of medicine" (1986:102) and warned that "as long as the medical profession tolerates that brand of infamy, the midwife, the public will not be brought to realize that there is high art in obstetrics and that it must pay as well for it as for surgery" (1986:105).

To convince the nation that obstetricians should replace midwives, physicians exaggerated the dangers and difficulty of childbirth, arguing "that no case is normal until it is over. At any moment complications are liable to arise capable of taxing the skill of the obstetrician to the utmost. In these emergencies, . . . unless a trained man is within easy reach the resulting delay means certain death for infant or mother, sometimes both" (Huntington, 1986:112). Loudly proclaiming the dangers of midwifery also helped to protect obstetricians' standing by providing scapegoats when turn-of-the-century social reformers began questioning high infant and maternal mortality rates in the United States compared to Europe (Dye, 1980:104).

Changes in the structure of medicine also pressured physicians to remove midwives as competition for poor as well as wealthier clients.

Only poor patients forced to go to lying-in charity hospitals could be used for the clinical research required by the new commitment to science. Middle- and upper-class women continued to be attended by physicians in the safer environments of their homes until almost mid-century, when use of sulfanilimide reduced the risk of puerperal sepsis. Hospitalized poor women also were needed to meet the growing demand for scientific training in clinical skills. One of the most active opponents of midwifery, Charles Ziegler, bemoaned the fact that "it is, at present, impossible to secure cases sufficient for the proper training of physicians, since 75 percent of the material otherwise available for clinical purposes is utilized in providing a livelihood for midwives" (1913:33).

Many prominent American obstetricians, particularly in Boston, argued for immediate eradication of midwives (Kobrin, 1984:320; Litoff, 1978:79–81). They considered any plan to regulate midwives a "great danger," since it might "giv[e] her thereby a legal status which later cannot perhaps be altered" (Ziegler, 1913:32). In their writings, these physicians described the midwife variously as "the typical, old, gin-fingering, guzzling midwife with her pockets full of forcing drops, her mouth full of snuff, her fingers full of dirt and her brains full of arrogance and superstition," "a relic of barbarism," "pestiliferous," "vicious," "ignorant, half-trained, [and] often malicious," "[with] the overconfidence of half-knowledge . . . unprincipled and callous of the feelings and welfare of her patients and anxious only for her fee" (quoted in Devitt, 1979a:89).

Physicians' arguments were strengthened by the marginal social and economic status of most turn-of-the-century midwives and their clients. In New York City, for example, only 4 percent of midwives practicing in 1906 were native-born Americans (Crowell, 1986:40). Physicians played on contemporary xenophobia, racism, and sexism in arguing that midwives were ignorant, uneducable, and a threat to true American values. For example, the director of the Mississippi Bureau of Child Hygiene, Dr. Felix J. Underwood, described black midwives as "filthy and ignorant and not far removed from the jungles of Africa, with its atmosphere of weird superstition and voodooism" (1926:683). The *Boston Medical and Surgical Journal* stressed the un-American nature of the immigrant midwives, who were "perhaps, an inevitable evil" in Europe but were "inconsistent with the

methods and ideals of civilization and of medical science in this country" (1915:785). As Wertz and Wertz describe, this attitude filtered
down to popular magazines which "treated immigrant midwives as
curious anachronisms, repeating horror stories replete with racial
and ethnic slurs about 'rat pie among black midwives' or deformed
babies allegedly delivered by Italian or Russian Jewish midwives"
(1977:216).

Opposition to midwifery was far from universal, however. Some
physicians, especially in the South, argued that midwives could not,
and should not, be eliminated even if they provided only second-class
care. These individuals recognized physicians' inability and unwillingness to service widely scattered rural populations, particularly
blacks and poor whites. In Mississippi, for example, midwives still
delivered about 90 percent of all black women in 1918 (Litoff,
1978:27).

Other physicians, notably in the New York area, supported the
New York Academy of Medicine's 1911 resolution promoting midwifery education and regulation (Jacobi, 1986:197). That same year,
an influential national survey of obstetrics professors found 18 in
favor of educating and regulating midwives compared to 14 favoring
total abolition (Williams, 1986:97), and New York City's health department opened a school for midwives at Bellevue Hospital. The
next year, Abraham Jacobi (1986) advocated midwifery licensing in
his presidential address to the AMA. The Pennsylvania State Bureau
of Medical Education responded and began model programs in midwifery education and supervision in 1914 (White House Conference
on Child Health and Protection, 1932). Maternal mortality among
the 90,926 cases attended by Philadelphia midwives over the next 16
years including those transferred to physicians was only 8 per 10,000.
In Pittsburgh it was 5, and in a group of ten rural counties it was 18.
In contrast the lowest recorded rate for the state as a whole during
these years, including physician attended births and abortions, was
61 per 10,000. Even when deaths from abortions are removed, the
state rate was still eight to nine times higher. Combined with similar
findings in New Jersey and even better findings in the population
served by the certified nurse-midwives of the Kentucky Frontier
Nursing Service, the Subcommittee on Obstetric Teaching and Education for the White House Conference on Child Health and Protec-

tion concluded that these statistics show "remarkably low rates for mothers attended by trained and supervised midwives" (1932:203).

Support for midwifery was particularly strong among public health physicians, who believed that trained midwives could be effective practitioners, that physicians could not meet the demand for assistance, and that many women were unable to afford physicians or unwilling to use them because of modesty (Kobrin, 1984:320). Midwives also retained support among those general practitioners who feared that if obstetricians successfully eradicated midwives, they might next focus their attention on removing competition from general practitioners (Litoff, 1978:103). Their fears were not baseless: in his survey, Williams found that most obstetrics professors believed general practitioners caused more needless deaths than did midwives, and concluded "why bother about the relatively innocuous midwife?" (1986:97).

Public health supporters of midwifery achieved their greatest success in 1921 with passage of the Sheppard–Towner Maternity and Infancy Protection Act (Lemons, 1973:153–80). Fourteen states chose to use funds provided under the act for midwifery training and regulatory programs. The act passed despite objections from the AMA and various conservative organizations that it heralded the start of socialized medicine and would reduce the quality of care (Lemons, 1973:159–66, 171–73; Wertz, 1983:22). Legislators had supported this and other social programs in a bid for votes after women won suffrage in 1920. The act's failure to gain renewal in 1929 reflected both the increased strength of the AMA and legislators' recognition that women had not become an important lobby (Lemons, 1973:157–58, 166, 174; Litoff, 1978:100; Wertz and Wertz, 1977:211).

While physicians' status was rising rapidly, their fight against midwives succeeded only partially in the legislative arena. By 1930, only Massachusetts, the center of the struggle, had outlawed midwifery (Litoff, 1986:9). Six states required only registration, and ten states neither licensed nor registered midwives. As Litoff notes, midwifery laws, while varied, were generally lenient and in some cases did not specify any penalties or were otherwise unforceable (1986:9–10). North Carolina, for example, only prohibited "drunkards and drug addicts" from practicing and required that those who practice for a fee "must wash and disinfect their hands" (White House Conference on Child Health and Protection, 1932:185). Typically, midwives were limited to normal births, prohibited from using drugs or instruments, and required to register all births and apply silver nitrate to the newborn's eyes. In certain jurisdictions, however, English literacy tests, examinations, or impossible education requirements did drive some midwives out of business (Anisef and Basson, 1979:367; Devitt, 1979b:181). Even "friendly" licensure inadvertently caused some to stop practicing, as officials in New York and New Jersey discovered (Litoff, 1986:9, 141).

Overall, legislation probably had a limited direct impact on midwives' numbers. Indirectly, however, by not upgrading the training and consequently the status of midwives, lenient legislation was a fatal blow to American midwifery. Concurrently, immigration restriction in the 1920s and the decline in birth rate during the Depression cut down both the demand for midwives and their supply (Devitt, 1979b:182). The use of physicians subsequently spread to the white working and lower classes. By the 1930s, midwives were disappearing outside the rural South and Southwest, where 80 percent worked (Reed, 1932). By 1935, midwives delivered 11 percent of American infants: 54 percent of nonwhite infants but only 5 percent of whites. By 1953, midwives delivered 3 percent of all births: fewer than 1 percent of white infants and 20 percent of nonwhites (Jacobson, 1956:254). With physician authority firmly established, the anti-midwifery campaign had long since ceased.

THE CONTRASTING FATE OF MIDWIVES IN EUROPE AND AMERICA

Unlike their American counterparts, European midwives continue to play a pivotal, although declining, role in health care (World Health Organization, 1985:80–81; 93–94). European midwives benefited from a long history of centralized control predating the growth in medical authority (Anisef and Basson, 1979:360–62; Devitt, 1979b:181; Donnison, 1977:1–41). Municipal regulation of midwives replaced ecclesiastical regulation in a few German and French communities as early as the fifteenth century and became widespread outside England during the sixteenth century. This evolved into state-sponsored regulation as nation-states formed.

With licensure came formal apprenticeship programs and public appointment of midwives to serve the poor. The first hospital-based training program opened at the famous Hotel Dieu in Paris in 1631. By the eighteenth century, several countries had begun similar state-subsidized programs for midwives. France further demonstrated its commitment to improving midwives' skills in 1770 by commissioning the king's physician to write a textbook for midwives and sponsoring a series of lectures for provincial midwives (Donnison, 1977:40). Education and examination of midwives eventually was placed under the control of the medical department of a university as in Denmark (White House Conference on Child Health and Protection, 1932:172).

In the capitalistic United States, in contrast, federal and local government rarely subsidized the training of any health care workers and few women could afford tuition (Arney, 1982:41; Donegan, 1984:310; Wertz and Wertz, 1977:44–45). The resulting financial risk severely limited interest in establishing proprietary training programs for midwives and left women with few if any opportunities for formal education.

Given the many educational programs available in continental Europe, physicians there could not reasonably disparage the quality of midwifery care. Furthermore, because of midwifery's status as a skilled, reputable occupation, it continued to attract educated middle-class women throughout the nineteenth century. New developments in obstetrical science were integrated into training programs and regulations tightened over time. By the end of the nineteenth century all European countries except England had public or private midwifery training programs varying from six months to three years in duration (White House Conference on Child Health and Protection, 1932:172). Whereas most European countries limited midwives to normal cases, Denmark and Sweden did not. None of the countries required that midwives' clients be screened by physicians, and France had no provision for supervision of their practices, giving French midwives complete autonomy. Thus, Continental midwives retained their social position into the twentieth century. English midwives, on the other hand, saw their occupational status decline with the waning power of the Church and the absence of other, rigorous regulation during the eighteenth and nineteenth centuries. They were rescued

from the brink of extinction by late nineteenth-century social reformers concerned about the plight of women (see chap. 9 for further discussion). These women had far greater resources—money,
central organization, power, and skills—than their American con-
temporaries when they began to fight for midwifery licensure in the
late nineteenth century. Moreover, they had a strong, centralized
government to lobby.

European midwives also fared better than American midwives because they faced less opposition from physicians (Anisef and Basson,
1979:358–59; Arney, 1982:40; Wertz and Wertz, 1977:48, 72). Physicians in Europe did not need to denigrate midwives in order to
increase their own social standing. European medical training was
far more advanced, and obtaining a medical education and license
considerably more difficult, than in the United States until at least
1910. European physicians enjoyed an elite status because of both
their training and their upper-class backgrounds. The obstacles to
licensure resulted in substantially lower physician/patient ratios than
in the United States, which limited European physicians' economic
incentive to eliminate midwives. Instead, European physicians' interests were served best by defining childbirth as a natural event for
the "sturdy" working and lower classes whose business they did not
want, while retaining for themselves only the wealthy and those urban poor useful for medical research or training (Anisef and Basson,
1979:359; Donnison, 1977:85–115).

Unique demographic patterns additionally hampered American
midwives. Midwives everywhere depend for their clients on personal
reputation among local networks of women. Extensive geographic
mobility in the United States weakened those networks (Wertz and
Wertz, 1977:47, 72). Unlike the fairly homogeneous populations of
midwives in European countries, ethnic, racial, linguistic, and religious differences, as well as geographic dispersion and poverty,
isolated American midwives and worked against building effective
alliances or even recognition of common interests (Anisef and
Basson, 1979:362–69). The lack of a national-level battle over midwifery regulation fatally weakened midwives' ability to break this
isolation from one another and from potential supporters. Despite
their historic differences, American physicians united at the turn of
the century to upgrade medical training with science, reestablish

public recognition of the complexity of health care, and advance themselves as appropriate, knowledgeable, health care practitioners. This set the stage for the passage of midwifery licensure laws in the twentieth century.

CONSEQUENCES OF THE DEMISE OF MIDWIFERY IN THE UNITED STATES

Once physicians replaced midwives as the primary attendants at childbirth, mortality and morbidity rates actually rose (Antler and Fox, 1976; Devitt, 1979b:185; Leavitt, 1983:299–303; Wertz, 1983:20). The higher maternal mortality of the United States compared to every European nation except one was a matter of concern to the White House Conference on Child Health and Protection in 1932. In all these countries except Scotland, more than one-half, and generally more than 80 percent, of births were attended by midwives. Contemporary studies attributed these differences to unnecessary and inept medical intervention, such as forceps deliveries, cesarean sections, and manual removal of the placenta, made possible by the new anesthetics and analgesics and frequently performed by general practitioners (Frankel, 1927; Levy, 1923; New York Academy of Medicine, 1933; White House Conference on Child Health and Protection, 1933). Yet physicians' skills had improved significantly in the United States since the Flexner Report pressured schools already threatened by increased costs and declining enrollment to tighten standards or close (Starr, 1982:118).

The upgrading of medical training increased admission standards, length of training, and, most important, costs. This left almost no schools which accepted blacks, women, or working-class students. As a result, attendance at childbirth not only moved from midwives to physicians but also from female to upper-class, white, male control.

Simultaneous with the final push to eradicate traditional midwives, however, the first moves were made toward establishing the new occupation of nurse-midwifery. The first school in which registered nurses could obtain advanced training in midwifery opened in 1925. Its founder, Mary Breckenridge, an American nurse who had trained as a midwife in England, established the Frontier Nursing Service to aid Kentucky's rural poor. Seven years later, the Maternity Center Association opened to serve New York City's urban poor.

These two organizations were the only sources of nurse-midwives for many years.

This new occupation did not expand significantly until the 1950s, when health officials faced a critical shortage of physicians. To reduce physicians' burdensome caseloads, several prestigious universities began training nurse-midwives to be "physician extenders." Nurse-midwives were expected to assume responsibility for normal births, which physicians considered routine, uninteresting, and unrenumerative, and to work for bureaucratic organizations serving poor and rural areas. The American College of Nurse-Midwives has certified 2,550 nurse-midwives since its establishment in 1955, of whom approximately 1,500 are currently practicing (American College of Nurse-Midwives, 1984:3–4). The college has cultivated carefully the support of the American College of Obstetrics and Gynecology. The former consistently describes nurse-midwives in its literature as members of the obstetric team, and "not independent practitioners" (Rothman, 1982:64–66). By accepting subordination, nurse-midwives have yielded midwives' traditional occupational territory to physicians.

MEDICALIZATION: THE SELLING OF SCIENCE

Physicians' success in taking over maternity care in the absence of clear evidence of better outcomes is one example of the broader expansion of medical authority that has characterized the twentieth century. This wider success ultimately rests upon the increase of 27 years in life expectancy between 1900 and 1983 (National Center for Health Statistics, 1984:53). Each new development of medical science—vaccinations, X rays, antibiotics, insulin therapy, chemotherapy, open heart surgery, organ transplants, in vitro fertilization, and the like—has been heralded by the media as a wondrous example of scientific ingenuity. Newspapers and magazines have columns devoted to informing readers about the newest medical developments, while television presents special programs on these innovations as well as incorporating them into general programming story-lines. This socialization has popularized the view that medical science, rather than the more crucial improvements in living conditions, is responsible for increased life expectancy (McKinlay and McKinlay, 1977); the rise in the gross national product does not have the dramatic appeal of an artificial heart.

As public confidence in medicine has grown, physicians have become the accepted experts in areas far beyond physiology. A wide range of situations and behaviors has been "medicalized," defined as diseases requiring skilled, scientific, medical intervention (Conrad and Schneider, 1980; Zola, 1972). Unhappy, menopausal women are labeled as sick with a hormonal deficiency disease, unruly children are diagnosed as "hyperactive," and persons who would have been considered sinners or criminals in previous eras are now defined as mentally ill. We turn to physicians for advice on everything from diet to love, child molestation to irregularity.

Both social scientists and consumer activists have called attention to the potential dangers inherent in medicalization (Conrad and Schneider, 1980; Zola, 1972). Medicalization can help individuals by reducing the stigma of sin but may replace it with the stigma of mental or physical illness. While some individuals gain access to beneficial treatment, in other cases medical and governmental authorities force questionable treatments on unwilling patients whose only "disease" may be unconventionality. "Sickness" provides some individuals a socially acceptable means of avoiding unpleasant work but in other instances allows physicians to restrict a "disabled" individual's activities against his or her will. Finally, medicalization encourages the public to trust physicians implicitly and to believe that only physicians are capable of making crucial decisions in an ever-expanding range of areas. This authority has led to unnecessary, costly, and risky interventions such as the excessive number of tonsillectomies in the postwar years and the more recent proliferation of radical mastectomies, hysterectomies, cesarean sections, and coronary bypass surgeries adopted by the public and the medical world without adequate prior evaluation (Millman, 1978:215–52). This authority also has brought psychiatrists into our courtrooms as experts on such deviant behaviors as premenstrual violence.

Awareness of the limits of medical science and the potential abuses inherent in intemperate medicalization has led to a recent backlash from a few consumers who have organized groups ranging from the National Women's Health Network to the Mental Patients Liberation Front (Starr, 1982:390–93). Whereas most parturient women initially welcomed medicine's increasing role in maternity care, the last several decades have seen the emergence of significant consumer dissatisfaction.

REFERENCES

American College of Nurse-Midwives. *Nurse-midwifery in the United States: 1982.* Washington, DC, 1984.

Anisef, Paul, and Priscilla Basson. "The institutionalization of a profession: A comparison of British and American midwifery." *Sociology of Work and Occupations* 6:353–72, 1979.

Antler, Joyce, and Daniel M. Fox. "The movement toward a safe maternity: Physician accountability in New York City, 1915–1940." *Bulletin of the History of Medicine* 50:569–95, Winter 1976.

Arney, William R. *Power and the Profession of Obstetrics.* Chicago: University of Chicago Press, 1982.

Bogdan, Jane. "Care or cure? Childbirth practices in nineteenth century America." *Feminist Studies* 4:92–99, 1978.

Boston Medical and Surgical Journal. "The midwife versus the pregnancy clinic." 173:784–85, 1915.

Conrad, Peter, and Joseph W. Schneider. *Deviance and Medicalization.* St. Louis: C. V. Mosby, 1980.

Crowell, F. Elizabeth. "The Midwives of New York," pp. 36–49 in Judy B. Litoff (ed.), *The American Midwife Debate.* Westport, CT: Greenwood Press, 1986.

De Lee, Joseph B. "Progress toward ideal obstetrics," pp. 102–09 in Judy B. Litoff (ed.), *The American Midwife Debates.* Westport, CT: Greenwood Press, 1986.

Devitt, Neal. "The transition from home to hospital birth in the United States, 1930–1960." *Birth and the Family Journal* 4:47–58, Summer 1977.

Devitt, Neal. "The statistical case for elimination of the midwife: Fact versus prejudice, 1890–1935" (Part 1). *Women and Health* 4:81–96, Spring 1979[a].

Devitt, Neal. "The statistical case for elimination of the midwife: Fact versus prejudice, 1890–1935" (Part 2). *Women and Health* 4:169–86. Summer 1979[b].

Donegan, Jane B. *Women and Men Midwives: Medicine, Morality, and Misogyny in Early America.* Westport, CT: Greenwood Press, 1978.

Donegan, Jane B. " 'Safe delivered,' but by whom?: Midwives and men midwives in early America," pp. 302–17 in Judith W. Leavitt (ed.), *Women and Health in America.* Madison: University of Wisconsin Press, 1984.

Donnison, Jean. *Midwives and Medical Men: History of Inter-Professional Rivalries and Women's Rights.* London: Heinemann, 1977.

Dye, Nancy S. "Review essay: History of childbirth in America." *Signs* 6 (1):97–108, 1980.

Ehrenreich, Barbara, and Deidre English. *Witches, Midwives and Nurses.* Old Westbury, NY: Feminist Press, 1973.

Forbes, Thomas R. *The Midwife and the Witch.* New Haven: Yale University Press, 1966.

Frankel, L. K. "The present status of maternal and infant hygiene in the United States." *American Journal of Public Health* 17:1909–39, 1927.

Gregory, Samuel. *Man-Midwifery Exposed and Corrected.* Boston: George Gregory, 1848.

Huntington, James L. "The midwife in Massachusetts: Her anomalous position," pp. 110–16 in Judy B. Litoff (ed.), *The American Midwife Debate.* Westport, CT: Greenwood Press, 1986.

Jacobi, Abraham. "The best means of combatting infant mortality," pp. 177–99 in Judy B. Litoff (ed.), *The American Midwife Debate.* Westport, CT: Greenwood Press, 1986.

Jacobson, P. H. "Hospital care and the vanishing midwife." *Milbank Memorial Fund Quarterly* 34:253–61, 1956.

Kobrin, Frances E. "The American midwife controversy: A crisis of professionalization," pp. 318–26 in Judith W. Leavitt (ed.), *Women and Health in America.* Madison: University of Wisconsin Press, 1984.

Leavitt, Judith W. " 'Science' enters the birthing room: Obstetrics in America since the eighteenth century." *Journal of American History* 70:281–304, 1983.

Leavitt, Judith W. *Brought to Bed: Childbearing in America, 1750–1950.* New York: Oxford University Press, 1986.

Lemons, J. Stanley. *The Woman Citizen: Social Feminism in the 1920s.* Urbana: University of Illinois Press, 1973.

Levy, Julius. "Maternal mortality and mortality in the first month in relation to attendant at birth." *American Journal of Public Health* 13:88-95, 1923.

Litoff, Judy B. *American Midwives: 1860 to the Present.* Westport, CT: Greenwood Press, 1978.

Litoff, Judy B. (ed.). *The American Midwife Debate.* Westport, CT: Greenwood Press, 1986.

McKinlay, John B., and Sonja J. McKinlay. "The questionable contribution of medical measures to the decline of mortality in the United States in the twentieth century." *Milbank Memorial Fund Quarterly* 55:405–28, Summer 1977.

Meigs, Charles D. *Females and Their Diseases: A Series of Letters to His Class.* Philadelphia, 1848.

Millman, Marcia. *The Unkindest Cut: Life in the Backrooms of Medicine.* New York: William Morrow, 1978.

National Center for Health Statistics. *Health, United States, 1984,* DHHS Pub. No. (PHS) 85-1232. Washington, DC: U.S. Government Printing Office, 1984.

National Center for Health Statistics. "Advance report of final natality statistics, 1983." *Monthly Vital Statistics Report* 34 (6), supplement September 20, 1985.

New York Academy of Medicine. *Maternal Mortality in New York City*. New York: Commonwealth Fund, 1933.

Population Reports. "Traditional Midwives and Family Planning." 8 (3): May 1980.

Quackenbush, John V. P. *An Address Delivered Before the Students of the Albany Medical College, Introductory to the Course on Obstetrics, November 5, 1855*. Albany, NY: B. Taylor, 1855.

Reed, L. *The Costs of Medicine: Midwives, Chiropodists, and Optometrists*. Chicago: University of Chicago Press, 1932.

Rothman, Barbara K. *In Labor: Women and Power in the Birthplace*. New York: Norton, 1982.

Scholten, Catherine. " 'On the importance of the obstetrick art': Changing customs of childbirth in America, 1760–1825," pp. 142–54 in Judith W. Leavitt (ed.), *Women and Health in America*. Madison: University of Wisconsin Press, 1984.

Semmelweis, Ignaz. *The Etiology, Concept, and Prophylaxis of Childbed Fever*. Madison: University of Wisconsin Press, 1983.

Starr, Paul. *The Social Transformation of American Medicine*. New York: Basic Books, 1982.

Underwood, Felix J. "Development of midwifery in Mississippi." *Southern Medical Journal* 19:683–85, 1926.

Welter, Barbara. "The cult of true womanhood: 1820–1860." *American Quarterly* 18:162–84, Summer 1966.

Wertz, Dorothy C. "What birth has done for doctors: A historical view." *Women and Health* 8 (1):7–24, Spring 1983.

Wertz, Richard W., and Dorothy C. Wertz. *Lying-In: A History of Childbirth in America*. New York: Free Press, 1977.

White House Conference on Child Health and Protection. *Obstetric Education*. New York: The Century Co., 1932.

White House Conference on Child Health and Protection. *Fetal, Newborn, and Maternal Mortality and Morbidity*. New York, 1933.

Williams, J. W. "Medical education and the midwife problem in the United States," pp. 86–101 in Judy B. Litoff (ed.), *The American Midwife Debate*. Westport, CT: Greenwood Press, 1986.

World Health Organization. *Having a Baby in Europe*. Public Health in Europe 26. Denmark, 1985.

Ziegler, Charles. "The elimination of midwives." *Journal of the American Medical Association* 60:32–38, 1913.

Zola, Irving K. "Medicine as an institution of social control." *Sociological Review* 20:487–504, 1972.

CHAPTER 2
THE REVOLT AGAINST
MEDICALIZED BIRTH

The elimination of midwifery and home birth was supposed to herald a new and better era for mothers and infants. No longer would women labor and deliver in unsanitary surroundings attended by uneducated midwives who could do little to relieve their pain, shorten their ordeal, or treat their complications. No longer would almost 1 percent of women and more than 4 percent of infants die from childbirth as at the turn of the century (U.S. Bureau of the Census, 1975:57). Instead, births would be actively managed with an ever expanding array of medical technologies and skills. Yet rather than wholeheartedly welcoming the medicalization of childbirth, a consumer movement, begun by a few dissatisfied parents in the 1950s, gained sufficient public support over the next two decades to challenge the medical model of childbirth. This chapter describes the reasons for this consumer movement and for its radical offshoot that advocates midwife-attended home birth.

HOSPITAL BIRTH IN THE MID-TWENTIETH CENTURY

The first half of the twentieth century witnessed a rapid increase in medical control of childbirth. Not only did birthing move from midwives to physicians but also from home to hospital. Whereas in 1900 fewer than 5 percent of births occurred in hospitals, by 1939 this proportion had multiplied tenfold (Wertz and Wertz, 1977:133), reaching 88 percent by 1950 (Devitt, 1977:56).

The shift from home to hospital caused significant changes in the nature of the childbirth experience. In the bureaucratic setting of the hospital women could no longer receive the individualized, personal care that had accompanied home birth among family and friends. Instead, new childbirth routines developed, not all of which were welcomed. Consumer dissatisfaction was demonstrated vividly in 1957 when the *Ladies Home Journal* published a letter from a registered nurse asking it "to investigate the tortures that go on in modern delivery rooms." The writer claimed that a mother-to-be is "strapped down with cuffs around her arms and legs and steel clamps over her shoulders and chest . . . with knees pulled far apart for as long as eight hours" (Shultz, 1958a:45). The voluminous response from readers outstripped that generated by even the most popular previous feature article, and supported the writer's accusations by a ratio of seven to one (Shultz, 1958b:45, 59). One wrote, for example: "I was strapped to the delivery table on Saturday morning and lay there until I was delivered on Sunday afternoon; [*sic*] with the exception of a period early Sunday morning when they needed the delivery table for an unexpected birth" (Schultz, 1958b:59). Another said: "My lips parched and cracked but the nurses refused to even moisten them with a damp cloth. I was left alone all night in a labor room. I felt exactly like a trapped animal and I am sure I would have committed suicide if I had had the means. Never have I needed someone, anyone, as desperately as I needed that night" (Schultz, 1958a:153). Experiences such as these led about 90 percent of the *Journal's* maternal correspondents to urge that hospitals allow husbands in labor and delivery rooms. One mother wrote, "Let them watch what goes on there. That's all it will take—they'll change it" (Schultz, 1958a:44).

While some nurses and doctors wrote to deny that any "tortures" take place in hospital labor and delivery, an equal number wrote to confirm the allegations. One nurse of thirty years added that she had "seen patients with no skin on their wrists from fighting the straps" (Shultz, 1958a:44). Those who denied the accusations of cruelty justified their actions by arguing that women had to be strapped down "to prevent contamination of the sterile field"; that steel shoulder braces were needed "for the mother's protection" (Shultz, 1958a:152); "that many women are spoiled, hysterical and full of fears; that most husbands are too emotionally unstable to stay with their wives during labor; that the memory of a childbirth experience is unreliable because of anesthetic drugs; [and] that there is simply not enough hospital and medical staff to give women the kind of care they seem to demand" (Shultz, 1958b:59).

Half the mothers who wrote to the *Journal* also complained that their deliveries were artificially slowed to await the physicians' arrival. Women told of nurses who tied their legs together, laid across them, or pushed against their babies' emerging heads to delay delivery until their physicians arrived. Leading obstetricians consulted by the *Journal* considered these procedures unnecessarily dangerous except in extreme circumstances because of the risk of fetal oxygen deprivation. A few mothers blamed their children's learning disabilities and perinatal deaths on such procedures.

Other women told of problems caused by induction or augmentation of labor. Like "hold back" procedures, elective induction was strongly condemned by the *Journal*'s medical consultants due to the risks of prematurity, uterine spasm, and oxygen deprivation. A registered nurse responding to the *Journal* letter described the tragedy that can result when labor is hastened without caution: "The mother . . . wasn't progressing fast enough to suit [her physician]. So he administered Pituitrin. . . . Before the cervix was completely dilated he put on forceps . . . to help things along. Then he proceeded to pull at the baby's head and—horror of horrors—the forceps slipped off twice. . . . The baby died of damage to the brain" (Shultz, 1958b:138). Despite such dangers, elective inductions were becoming increasingly common; popular articles discussing the advantages of "Babies by Appointment" appeared in both *McCalls* and *Reader's Digest* in 1957.

Other hospital practices to which the *Journal*'s readers objected had been introduced because of the need to control puerperal fever in the germ-laden hospital environment. Sulfa drugs, introduced in the 1940s, and penicillin in later years reduced this threat. As a result, douches and kerosene scrubs are no longer used. However, antiseptic and aseptic measures, including a few with questionable utility, remain part of the hospital routine. Women are given enemas, partially shaved in the pubic area, moved to aseptic rooms for delivery, scrubbed, and draped. In addition, women and newborns were, and sometimes still are, isolated from their families and each other to avoid contamination. As recently as the 1970s, parental contact with newborns was generally limited to "a glimpse of the baby at birth, a brief contact for identification at 6 to 8 hours, and then visits of 20 to 30 minutes for feeding every 4 hours" (Klaus and Kennell, 1976:54). Such rules can seem capricious, as one mother described: "I couldn't touch my baby for three days. He was in isolation in case there'd been an infection in utero. It was crazy! I had my baby and they took him away and I couldn't touch him. Then we went home. As I was leaving, they put me in a wheelchair, plopped the baby in my lap, and pushed me out of the hospital" (Arms, 1975a:21).

In addition to distressing many women who viewed antiseptic practices as arbitrary and excessive, these procedures had a major side effect on infant nutrition. The limited interaction between mothers and babies and the rigid feeding schedules designed to fit bureaucratic routine during the average six-day hospital stay in 1951 (U.S. Public Health Service, 1964) made breastfeeding difficult to establish. The prevailing medical view of a mother's breast as a potential souce of dangerous germs further compounded the problem. Many maternity staffs used a precautionary alcohol wash which aggravated the tendency of a new nursing mother's nipples to dry, crack, and bleed. This common problem limited women's desire and ability to breastfeed. As an alternative, doctors prescribed sterilized "formulas" to be given on fixed schedules suitable for hospital routine.

Infant formulas first attracted medical attention in the 1870s but remained controversial and difficult to prepare until pasteurized commercial mixes appeared in the late 1920s. Pharmaceutical companies marketed these products as social and nutritional improvements over mother's milk. Bottle feeding enhanced the social status of women by giving them freedom previously enjoyed only by those who could afford wet nurses. Moreover, as mothers monitored the ounces of formula consumed, they could feel confident that their babies were getting enough of the very best nutrition modern science had to offer. In an era of "better living through science," bottle-feeding, like the washing machine, garbage disposal, and other new technologies, was rapidly adopted; by 1972 only 21 percent of women were breastfeeding at discharge (Meyer, 1958:117) compared to more than 90 percent in 1922 (Woodbury, 1922:669).

Like antiseptic practices, pain control technology also proliferated. The chloroform and ether that nineteenth-century physicians had used to dull pain gave way to newer and more powerful drugs (Wertz and Wertz, 1977:118). The most popular was Twilight Sleep, a combination of morphine and scopolamine, an amnesic which erases the memory of pain (Sandelowski, 1984:3–26). When concern about scopolamine-caused hallucinations and agitation and the hazards of narcotics grew in the 1950s, it was gradually replaced by newer anesthetics and analgesics (Sandelowski, 1984:28–31, 93). These, too, entailed some risk and had consequences for the nature of maternity care beyond the vomiting and headaches that often resulted and the rare but vexing maternal deaths.

The increased use of analgesics and anesthetics fostered a rise in operative interventions. Not only did anesthetics and analgesics make surgery a safer and hence more attractive option when complications arose, they also increased the need for interventions because they diminished uterine contractions and women's ability to push during delivery. To offset this undesirable side effect, physicians increasingly resorted to other drugs to stimulate uterine contractions. Many also heeded the advice of Dr. Joseph B. De Lee (1920) and began routinely using forceps and episiotomies, procedures which earlier physicians had used only in emergencies.[1]

Physicians justified the psychological and physical discomforts of hospital childbirth by the trend in improved outcomes; maternal mortality had fallen from 61 per 10,000 in 1915 to 8 in 1950, while neonatal deaths declined over the same period from 44 per 1,000 to 20 (U.S. Bureau of the Census, 1975:57). Nevertheless, some consumers began to question whether all the routines developed as part of the active medical management of childbirth were necessary, and regarded some, especially isolating family members, as extreme.

1. No national statistics were kept on these procedures prior to 1979, so it is impossible to ascertain the exact rates. Some indications of the situation can be derived from studies such as that conducted at the innovative "natural childbirth" program at Yale, where physicians in 1949–50 used forceps with 16 percent and episiotomies with 87 percent of women having their first babies (Thoms and Wyatt, 1951:207–08). Similarly, O'Leary and O'Leary (1965) mentioned without comment or justification a 95 percent episiotomy rate in their practice between 1954 and 1964.

This discontent gained support from the postwar glorification of family values and motherhood as women's most important role. As other life options narrowed, women increasingly sought gratification from childbirth, as well as from childrearing and domesticity (Sandelowski, 1984:75, 113–15; Wertz and Wertz, 1977:183–90). Consequently, a growing number of women in the 1950s wanted to stay "awake and aware" in order to enjoy the "spiritual experience" of giving birth.

THE RISE OF CHILDBIRTH CONSUMER GROUPS

The first attack on modern childbirth practices came from Grantly Dick-Read, a British obstetrician (1944).[2] Read castigated physicians for neglecting women's subjective experience of childbirth, and argued that physicians' view of pregnant women as malfunctioning machines had interfered with the natural birthing process, producing fear, tension, and, consequently, pain in women. To keep women relaxed and unafraid, he proposed that physicians educate women in the normal, healthy physiology of childbearing; allow husbands or other supportive individuals to accompany women during labor and delivery; recognize the importance of psychological factors in childbirth; and respond to patients' individual desires. Read's influence grew slowly after he visited the United States in 1947 on a speaking tour sponsored by the Maternity Center Association. A number of popular magazines gave Read's views visibility in the 1950s, including *Ladies Home Journal,* which published a condensation of his book in 1957. Childbirth education groups based on his ideas subsequently sprang up in this country, leading to the formation of the International Childbirth Education Association (ICEA) in 1960. The organization had grown to 11,500 individual members in 31 countries by 1984.

A second challenge to contemporary maternity care practices came from Soviet physicians who in the 1950s used Pavlovian conditioning techniques to desensitize women to childbirth pain. Their "psycho-

2. Read's book was published under the title *Natural Childbirth* in 1933 in London (Heinemann) but did not reach the United States until 1944; the hyphenated version of his name is rarely used in the United States.

prophylactic method" taught women to respond to uterine contractions with relaxation, structured breathing patterns, and muscular control rather than with fear, tension, and pain. Its originators hoped to enable women to avoid analgesia and anesthesia. A French doctor, Fernand Lamaze, introduced these ideas to Western Europe in 1958. They became known to American audiences through the book *Thank You, Dr. Lamaze: A Mother's Experience in Painless Childbirth* (Karmel, 1959), written by an American woman who had given birth in Lamaze's French clinic. Its author, Marjorie Karmel, founded the American Society for Psychoprophylaxis in Obstetrics (ASPO) in 1960 to provide labor coaches and prepare women for childbirth. When demand exceeded the availability of trained coaches, the ASPO modified the Lamaze approach and began training husbands and significant others to fill this role. There were 10,000 Lamaze instructors by 1986 (Lesko, 1986:123), up from 320 in 1969 (Gurney, 1973:154).

Over the years numerous other childbirth education groups were established. Each method—Bradley, Harris, Gamper—gained adherents to its own, somewhat different approach. All these groups, however, shared a basic belief in the naturalness of childbirth.

As challenges to the medical model of childbirth gained strength, some mothers also began to question accepted medical wisdom on the superiority of infant formula, rigid feeding schedules, and early introduction of solid food over more "natural" feeding practices. This subsidiary attack on medical authority came to a head in 1956, when seven mothers formed La Leche League to aid other women who wanted to breastfeed. In an era in which the feminine mystique flourished, the league found a ready and sympathetic audience for its promotion of breastfeeding as a natural, superior, and "womanly" method. La Leche continues to help women who want to breastfeed by providing practical information through meetings, newsletters, and its book, *The Womanly Art of Breastfeeding* (La Leche League International, 1958). More important, the league provides emotional support and bolsters the confidence of women who encounter opposition to breastfeeding from family, friends, and physicians. The league now has about 30,000 members in this country (personal communication, 10/22/86), compared to 17,000 in 1970 (Newsweek, 1970a:63).

Increasing numbers of consumers also began to question the pregnancy diets recommended by their physicians. These diets were designed to limit weight gain to less than twenty pounds. Physicians
argued that the restricted weight gain would ease delivery and reduce the risk of toxemia, a potentially fatal complication of pregnancy characterized by fluid retention, high blood pressure, and protein
in the urine. Many women had a difficult time adhering to the prescribed diets and resented being chastised and patronized during
prenatal visits for their weight gain. Although this discontent never
sparked a separate consumer organization, it did fuel the larger dissatisfaction with contemporary maternity care.

Proposals for natural or prepared childbirth, admitting fathers
into delivery rooms, keeping mothers and babies together, breast-
feeding, and other changes disturbed physicians by threatening to
draw childbearing women into the decision-making process (Sandelowski, 1984:131–32). A woman who understands her physiology
and has someone to support and articulate her choices about childbirth procedures is far more likely to assert her preferences. Similarly, the consumer groups challenged physicians' power not because
they promoted drugless childbirth, family bonding, or breastfeeding
but because they encouraged mothers to trust their own and other
mothers' thoughts and feelings about childbirth and infants' needs.
As a result, women who wanted these alternatives met significant
hostility from physicians, frequently finding themselves branded as
"trouble-makers." One physician, quoted in *Newsweek* (1965:98),
called them a "compulsive-neurotic group" in "Oxford shoes" who
"write down exactly what you tell them." Another physician and his
coauthor denounced the movement's "un-American" origins in the
Soviet Union and England as a threat to democracy and womankind
(Fielding and Benjamin, 1962a) and published the "Medical Case
against Natural Childbirth" in *McCalls* (1962b) to lobby for women's
support.

More effective and more common than these overt attacks or de-
fensive claims from physicians that "natural childbirth is for women
in rice paddies" (*Newsweek*, 1965:98), were numerous articles written
by physicians for women's magazines explaining and rationalizing
the routinized obstetrical practices of episiotomy, forceps, sedation,
and exclusion of fathers and other intimates from labor and delivery

(for example, Gerbie, 1967; Gorbach, 1972). This subtle campaign, combined with the influence exerted by women's personal physicians, created a major obstacle to change.

GATHERING SUPPORT FOR ALTERNATIVES

Advocates of maternity care reform, including some physicians, sought to overcome resistance with a wealth of scientific studies documenting the problems with standard medical practices. Supporters of natural childbirth education conducted numerous studies comparing the outcomes of trained and untrained mothers (reviewed in Hughey et al., 1978). Although Beck (1978) argues that most of these studies suffer from methodological flaws, the findings consistently indicated that women trained in psychoprophylactic techniques had shorter labors, lost less blood, required less anesthesia and analgesia and fewer operative interventions, produced happier and healthier babies, and experienced greater personal satisfaction. Other medical research demonstrated that pain relief drugs given to mothers passed through the placenta and adversely affected infants at least temporarily. In the absence of research documenting the long-term impact of drug use, in 1978 the American Academy of Pediatrics in consultation with the American College of Obstetrics and Gynecology recommended keeping drug use to a minimum during labor and delivery (Committee on Drugs, 1978). In light of these developments, even those obstetricians most hostile to childbirth education had to acknowledge the positive benefits of decreased medication, especially anesthesia, which can severely lower blood pressure and diminish uterine contractions. The change in physicians' attitudes about childbirth education might also have been helped by the realization that women who had taken childbirth classes and had a support person present were calmer and more compliant than other patients (Rothman, 1981:169).

Concern about delivery procedures also led to research on the effects of different positions for giving birth. The accepted lithotomy position, in which the woman lies on her back, allowed the physician to assume a more comfortable and dignified posture with a good view of the birth. At the same time, however, it forced women to work against gravity. Consequently, as various studies (reviewed in

Roberts, 1980a, 1980b) demonstrated, the lithotomy position significantly increased the difficulty of delivering for many mothers, resulting in increased pain and perineal lacerations. In addition, this position constricted women's blood vessels, resulting in decreased blood
flow to the uterus and the potential for fetal oxygen deprivation.
These studies led Roberto Caldeyro-Barcia, then president of the
International Federation of Gynecologists and Obstetricians, to label
lithotomy the "worst position" for labor and delivery (1975).

Other researchers studied the potential hazards of induction,
whether through breaking the amniotic membrane or through administering drugs to start labor contractions. While many argued
that the benefits of preventing postmaturity and toxemia far out-
weighed the dangers, (Cole et al., 1975; Martin et al., 1978; Clinch,
1979; Miles, 1951; Reycraft, 1951; British Medical Journal, 1972;
O'Driscoll et al., 1969; O'Driscoll et al., 1973; McNay et al., 1977;
Pearce et al., 1979; Lancet, 1982; Husbands, 1950; Erving and Kenwick, 1952), the reformers took a dimmer view. Induction, they observed, produces stronger, more painful contractions than natural
labor. These stronger contractions can damage the soft bones of
infants' skulls, cut off infants' oxygen supply by compressing the
umbilical cord, and rupture women's uteri (Baumgarten, 1976;
Fields, 1960; Lynaugh, 1980; Caldeyro-Barcia, 1975; Blaikley, 1956;
Wilson, 1953; Claman et al., 1984; Yudkin et al., 1979; Liston and
Campbell, 1974). Because of the added pain, induction results in
greater use of drugs, with concommitant dangers (Yudkin et al.,
1979; Martin et al., 1978; Ingemarsson et al., 1981; Smith et al.,
1984). Before medical techniques for dating pregnancies and caring
for preterm infants improved, induction could also lead to the delivery of premature babies, whose lungs were insufficiently developed
to prevent anoxia, brain damage, or even death (Lancet, 1974; Blacow
et al., 1975; British Medical Journal, 1970; Maisels et al., 1977; Chalmers et al., 1978). Finally, rupturing the membranes increases the
rate of infection for both mother and infant (Blaikley, 1956; Fields,
1960; Wilson, 1953; MacDonald, 1970) and the rate of infant jaundice (Chew and Swann, 1977; D'Souza et al., 1979; Chalmers et al.,
1975). Although these risks may be worth taking in emergencies,
they did not seem otherwise justified.

To counter the standard practice of separating mothers and

babies, childbirth activists pointed to the demonstrated importance in early animal studies of imprinting and the maternal-infant bond. The authors of subsequent studies on humans included fathers and siblings, as well as mothers, and argued that practices which limited family access to newborns interfered with the development of family ties during the critical first minutes or hours (Klaus and Kennell, 1976; Peterson and Mehl, 1977; de Chateau, 1977). Proponents argued with emotional, if not always scientific, persuasion that the lack of immediate contact with newborns contributes to divorce, child abuse, failure to thrive among infants, and emotional distance within families (Arney, 1982:160–65; Fraiberg, 1977; Palkovitz, 1982). By emphasizing the dangers of these "social diseases," activists gained support for their aims in the face of concern that such contact might increase the risk of infectious diseases.

Researchers also documented the advantages of breastfeeding over infant formulas. Studies suggested that breastfeeding provides better nutrition than formulas (Ahn and MacLean, 1980; Casey et al., 1981; Janas et al., 1985; Lubin et al., 1981; Picciano and Deering, 1980), particularly for preterm and low birth weight babies (Atkinson et al., 1983; Oberkotter et al., 1985; Gross and Gabriel, 1985); gives infants some protection against allergies, diseases, and possibly future obesity (Gerrard, 1974; Gyorgy et al., 1962; Hide and Guyer, 1985; Fallot et al., 1980; Lepage et al., 1981; Narayanan et al., 1980; Narayanan et al., 1981; Narayanan et al., 1984; Bullen and Willis, 1971; Murray, 1971; Winberg and Wessner, 1971; Cunningham, 1977; Cunningham, 1979; Yoshioka et al., 1983; Larsen and Homer, 1978; France et al., 1980; Kramer, 1981; Kramer et al., 1985; Warren et al., 1964; Downham et al., 1976; Persico et al., 1983; Myers et al., 1984; Forman et al., 1984; Ellestad-Sayed et al., 1979; Saarinen et al., 1979; Borch-Johnsen et al., 1984; Beerens et al., 1980; Hoyle et al., 1980) produces long-term psychological benefits for children (Aldrich, 1947; Hughes and Hawkins, 1975; Hughes and Bushnell, 1977); and offers mothers some protection against later breast cancer (Byers et al., 1985; Ing et al., 1977).

Other research suggested that restricting weight gain during pregnancy to less than 20 pounds increases infant mortality and morbidity by lowering the average birth weight (Singer et al., 1968). In 1970, the National Academy of Sciences recommended an average gain of 24 pounds (Committee on Maternal Nutrition, 1970); current obstetrical guidelines recommend weight gains of 22 to 27 pounds (American Academy of Pediatrics and the American College of Obstetrics and Gynecology, 1983). No national studies evaluating the impact of maternal weight gain were completed until 1986, however. In that year, a major study concluded that adequate weight gain could reduce the risk of fetal death by as much as 59 percent (National Center for Health Statistics, 1986:14).

As research findings in favor of changing maternity care practices mounted, more consumers, physicians, and nurses became involved with reform. The converted brought their new doctrine to the public through the classes and services they offered and through the media, especially women's magazines. In the years following the letter complaining about maternity care in *Ladies Home Journal*, articles advocating anesthesia (Anderson, 1965; Ostapowicz, 1971; Wylie, 1969) and extolling the conveniences of elective induction (*Good Housekeeping*, 1961; *McCalls*, 1957; *Reader's Digest*, 1957; *Newsweek*, 1970b), elective forceps (*Good Housekeeping*, 1965), bottle feeding (Smart, 1950), or the high technology of birthing in an abdominal decompression chamber (Mendels, 1963; *Time*, 1967; Yuncker, 1969) gradually were outnumbered by those promoting natural childbirth and childbirth education (Bing, 1976; Feinbloom, 1973; Grossman, 1959; Harris, 1956; Hoover, 1974; Kalkstein, 1971; *Parents Magazine*, 1971; Seligmann, 1976; Senn, 1963; Sensibar, 1969; Sutherland, 1974; *Time*, 1964; Williams, 1973), fathers in the delivery room (Goldfarb and Goldfarb, 1958; Marshall, 1974; Powers, 1974; Spero, 1965; Sutherland, 1974), breastfeeding (Wessel, 1965; *Saturday Evening Post*, 1979; Weber, 1979; Reuben, 1971; Lehrer, 1975; Kenyon, 1946; *Good Housekeeping*, 1963; *Newsweek*, 1970a; Riker, 1960; *Time*, 1965, 1968; Baker, 1963; Grace of Monaco, 1971; Spock, 1957; M. Clark, 1978; Carlson, 1973; Cranch, 1977; *Parents Magazine*, 1945; *Ladies Homes Journal*, 1975; Carro, 1978; O'Keefe, 1962; *Consumer Reports*, 1977; *Parents Magazine*, 1950; Rawlins, 1968; Shultz, 1955; Pryor, 1963; Henig, 1979; Carroll, 1947) and bonding (Brazelton, 1971; Harris, 1956; Longwell, 1966), and those discussing the hazards of induction, medication, and other hospital procedures (Arms, 1975a; Brazelton, 1971; Brenner and Brenner, 1966; Brody, 1975; Davidson, 1964; Lake, 1976; Nolen, 1971; Yuncker, 1975). Numerous popular books on childbirth alternatives appeared as well, including the ICEA president's influential *Cultural Warping of Childbirth* (Haire, 1972), *The Birth Book* (Lang, 1972), *Spiritual Midwifery* (Gaskin, 1975), *Immaculate Deception* (Arms, 1975b), and *The Rights of Pregnant Parents* (Elkins, 1976). By this time the Lamaze method was regarded as a "traditional alternative" (N. Clark, 1976) and Leboyer's radical proposal for "birth without violence" was enthusiastically reviewed in *Vogue* (Milinaire, 1974), *Ms.* (Torres, 1974), *Reader's Digest* (Schreiner, 1976), and *Newsweek* (Alexander, 1975).

THE EROSION OF MEDICAL AUTHORITY

Public receptivity to the reformers' advocated changes in maternity care was enhanced by changing social norms and values. The thalidomide tragedy of the early 1960s had undermined the social trust that the antibiotic "wonder drugs" of the 1940s had won for pharmaceutical companies. More generally, the civil rights movement, the antipoverty campaign, the Vietnam War, feminist activity, and environmental deterioration had bequeathed a skepticism about the righteousness of social institutions that cast a shadow over medicine as well as government, education, and industry. Out of the social turmoil—the study groups, protest marches, sit-ins, riots, lawsuits, legislation, utopian communes, and attempts to "find oneself"— came a new-found desire for a more moral, natural way of living. The strength of this new American value in the 1970s can be gauged by the phenomenal success of marketing strategies that promoted such diverse products as cosmetics and margarine as "natural," in spite of the oxymorons created in the process.

Studies of women who choose alternative childbirth options such as natural childbirth or breastfeeding find that they are disproportionately older, wealthier, and more educated than users of standard care (Cave, 1978; Cohen, 1982; Eakins, 1984; Koop and Brannon, 1984:553–54; Moran and von Bargen, 1982). Nevertheless, demand for alternatives has become widespread. By 1980, 54 percent of new mothers initiated breastfeeding (Martinez et al., 1981). A survey of all resident Arizonan women to whom a birth certificate was issued during one month in 1978 reported that almost all wanted to have a family member present, remain conscious, receive encouragement to use breathing and relaxation techniques, have the freedom to move around during labor, and stay with their newborn after birth (Sullivan and Beeman, 1981:156, 1982:327). More than half (58 percent) wanted to breastfeed. However, the same proportion still wanted pain medication during labor.

As childbirth alternatives gained public support in the 1970s, the cultural authority of physicians declined. The new public attitude is visible in the exponential increase in malpractice suits and the size of awards, especially for childbirth cases. Obstetrical insurance costs since the early 1980s are among the highest in medicine, leading 9 percent of obstetrician-gynecologists in 1983 to cease delivering babies rather than pay up to $83,000 for coverage (Casselberry, 1985:630).

Equally persuasive evidence of physicians' eroding authority can be seen in the federal government's decision to conduct studies of various obstetrical-gynecological practices. Although the government's involvement in these issues may derive as much from its new role as a third-party payer of Medicaid and Medicare bills as from its historic interest in public health, its authority, unlike that of consumer groups and lawyers, cannot be discounted easily by physicians.

Federal employees document that despite physicians' increasing verbal support for "natural childbirth" in the 1970s, the rate of cesarean deliveries continues to rise and stands at 20 percent in 1985 (Taffel et al., 1985) compared to 4 percent in 1965 (Banta and Thacker, 1979:245). In contrast, the World Health Organization (WHO) believes there is "no justification for a rate above 10 to 15 percent" (1985:437).

Physicians argue that the high cesarean rate stems from the reduced use of more dangerous high forceps, avoidance of difficult vaginal breech deliveries, and the need to practice defensively in a litigious society (Pearse, 1983). Researchers, however, point to other sources, beginning with the medical doctrine of "once a cesarean, always a cesarean." Yet a review of the obstetrical literature, sponsored by the government, finds no evidence that the small risk of uterine rupture in a vaginal birth following a cesarean justified applying such a rule to most women (U.S. Public Health Service, 1981:351–67).

Federal and private researchers also find that the adoption of electronic fetal monitoring technology has contributed to the rise in cesareans (Banta and Thacker, 1979; Leveno et al., 1986; U.S. Public Health Service, 1981:394–401). Monitoring machines provide a continuous record of labor and require less staff time than fetal stethoscopes. However, WHO recommends against their routine use (1985:437) because they are more prone to false readings of fetal distress, resulting in unnecessary cesareans.

Some radical critics such as Scully (1980) and Cohen and Estner (1983) additionally blame the rise of cesareans on physicians' greed and boredom with uncomplicated deliveries. As evidence they note that cesareans are more common among women with private physicians and better insurance coverage, despite their higher social status and, consequently, lower obstetrical risk (Haynes de Regt et al., 1986).

Other obstetrical and gynecological practices that came under special governmental scrutiny in the 1970s include amniocentesis, episiotomy, and hysterectomy. Research concluded that amniocentesis is "an accurate and highly safe procedure that does not add significant risk to the pregnancy" (NICHD National Registry for Amniocentesis Study Group, 1976:23). In contrast, a review of the medical literature finds no support for the routine episiotomies which are performed in nearly two-thirds of all deliveries (Banta and Thacker, 1982), and WHO recommends against routine use of this procedure (1985:437). Similarly, researchers question the legitimacy of some criteria used to justify elective hysterectomies. Dicker and associates (1982) find that only about one in ten are for cancer, uncontrollable postpartum hemorrhage, uterine rupture, or other life-threatening conditions. Included as justifications for some of the other elective surgeries are menstrual discomfort, sterilization, tipped uterus, small fibroids, and other minor health problems. Another group of researchers conclude that since "hysterectomy is often discretionary on medical grounds, . . . an opportunity is created for non-biological factors, such as the nature and extent of a woman's insurance coverage, to play a major role" (Koepsell et al., 1980:41). Perhaps as a result of the controversy created by the government's surveillance program and predictions that half of all American women would soon have their uteri removed if the mid-1970s' rate continued, the number of hysterectomies fell 10 percent but is once again increasing.

THE HOME BIRTH MOVEMENT

The government's findings have lent greater credibility to the growing childbirth consumer movement. New organizations have
formed, including the InterNational [*sic*] Association of Parents and
Professionals for Safe Alternatives in Childbirth (NAPSAC) and the
Cesarean Prevention Movement. The diverse consumer movement
has succeeded in changing many hospital obstetrical policies. In the
1980s women are no longer routinely strapped down for delivery or
shaved over the entire pubic area. Most hospitals finally allow fathers
and other intimates to remain during normal labor and delivery and
permit greater and more flexible contact between mothers and newborns. The latter has facilitated the increase in breastfeeding—officially proclaimed the preferred infant nutrition by WHO in 1974
(Twenty-seventh World Health Assembly) and by the Canadian
Paediatric Society and the American Academy of Pediatricians in
1978 (Nutrition Committee). The average hospital stay dropped to
only three days by 1984 (personal communication, National Center
for Health Statistics, 9/22/86). Many hospitals now offer 12- and 24-
hour early release plans following normal deliveries, reflecting a
growing recognition of childbirth as a natural, nonpathological
event.

In spite of these consumer victories, physicians retain control over
the childbirth process in the hospital. To deflect consumer disenchantment, the American Academy of Pediatrics, American College
of Nurse-Midwives, American College of Obstetricians and Gynecologists, and American Nurses' Association in 1978 published an official statement encouraging "family-centered maternity/newborn
care" (Interprofessional Task Force on Health Care of Women and
Children). Following this directive, most hospitals now offer their
own coopted version of childbirth education classes, aptly renamed
"childbirth preparation classes." These classes, usually taught by labor nurses, offer a "modified Lamaze Method" or the Harris Method. The key objective is to avoid conflict with hospital routines; the
Harris Method, for example, claims that it "lets the doctor practice
medicine" (Lesko, 1986:124). Instead of encouraging women to seek
information and participate actively in childbirth decisions and procedures, hospital-sponsored classes socialize women to expect and

accept hospital routines, including fetal monitors, intravenous drips, labor augmentation, forceps, analgesics during early labor, and anesthetics during delivery. Instructors tell women that they "shouldn't try to be heroes" and gloss over the side effects of medication. Women are psychologically prepared for a cesarean should their physician judge it appropriate.

Physicians also have retained control of childbirth by manipulating the definition of natural childbirth. Much like advertising executives promoting "natural" products, physicians see no contradiction in telling women that they had a natural birth even if their deliveries included induction, episiotomy, anesthesia, analgesics, and forceps (Wertz and Wertz, 1977:195–96; Sandelowski, 1984:97). The first American physicians who actively promoted natural childbirth reported that they used analgesia during vaginal births in 81 percent of women having their first births (nulliparas) and 52 percent of the rest, administered anesthetics in 69 and 55 percent, respectively, and cut epsiotomies in 87 and 22 percent, respectively (Thoms and Wyatt, 1951:207–08). Similarly, among Lamaze-trained women seen between 1969 and 1979 at the influential Manchester Memorial Hospital birthing center, 72 percent of nulliparas and 38 percent of the rest received an anesthetic during labor, whereas 43 and 23 percent, respectively, received an anesthetic during delivery (Sumner and Phillips, 1981:41–44).

By the late 1960s, an increasing number of women were strongly committed to and had prepared for a family-centered natural childbirth. They often suffered disappointment, however, when hospital staff, a substitute physician, or even their own personal physician overrode their choice and refused fathers entry to delivery, ordered heavier sedation and labor augmentation, or cut an episiotomy. Recognizing the limits on true reform within hospitals, the most disenchanted started choosing home birth. These individuals believe that they will never gain sufficient control within hospitals to replace the active medical management of a passive "diseased" patient with a more holistic, wellness model that stresses self-responsibility, family involvement, and minimal medical intervention. To promulgate their views, they formed groups such as Informed Homebirth, the Association for Childbirth at Home (ACAH), and Home Oriented Maternity Experience, Inc. (HOME) beginning in the early 1970s.

Although no rigorous studies are available, several motives emerge consistently in descriptions of couples who have chosen home birth. The existing research suggests that the choice of home birth may stem from a philosophy that defines childbirth as a normal process, stresses the importance of family, and emphasizes personal responsibility and control (Anderson et al., 1978; Cameron et al., 1979; Hazell, 1975; Searles, 1981). Hazell (1974, 1975) and Cameron et al. (1979) conclude that the home birth parents in California and Utah, respectively, differed significantly in philosophy but not in demographic background from others, whereas Dingley (1977, 1979) finds that women choosing home birth in Oregon are younger, more educated and have more children than others. Similarly, Mehl and Peterson (1976) conclude that home birth parents in California and Wisconsin are disproportionately upper middle class. Burnett and collegues find that the few who plan an unattended home birth in North Carolina are more likely than the state average to be over 20, white, married, and educated (1980:2744). Federal statistics do not differentiate between births at home and in freestanding birth centers, between planned and unplanned out-of-hospital deliveries, or between lay and certified nurse-midwives. Data for 1984 indicate that 39 percent of midwife-attended out-of-hospital births are to women aged 30 or above, and 50 percent are to women with some college education (National Center for Health Statistics, unpublished data); the comparable rates for hospital births are 24 percent and 36 percent, respectively (National Center for Health Statistics, 1986).

Financial considerations may also be important (Cameron et al., 1979) particularly in states where home birth midwifery is legal and hence more easily available (Weitz and Sullivan, 1985:50). Burnett and associates found that North Carolina women who chose home birth attended by a lay midwife were disproportionately young, black, unmarried, and with relatively little formal education (1980:2744). In 1984, 17 percent of reported births in homes and freestanding birthing centers occurred among immigrants, rising to 24 percent among those attended by lay or certified nurse-midwives (National Center for Health Statistics, unpublished data). Almost two-thirds (63 percent) of foreign-born women who gave birth out-of-hospital were Mexican-born, and 58 percent lived in Texas; 52 percent were Mexican-born Texas residents. Where these numbers reflect planned home births rather than accidental out-of-hospitals births or births at birthing centers, they represent the continuation of an older tradition based on economic necessity rather than philosophical choice.

For couples who view birth as a natural, safe event, the physical and psychological discomforts of hospital care seem best avoided, and surrendering decision-making to medical authorities seems an unwarranted loss of personal control. Most of these couples also feel that hospital birth eliminates an essential opportunity to strengthen family ties. One couple explains their choice:

> Foremost, and underlying our whole enthusiasm for homebirth, was our desire to be in control of the situation. The setting was familiar and comfortable. We could arrange it to suit our needs. Instead of us being "intruders" into the medical personnels' world, the midwife and the doctor were visitors. During the process of labor we were freed from having to respond to new and unfamiliar hospital routines and [having] to adjust ourselves to conform to the behavioral expectations of others. . . .
>
> We [Martha and Bill] were able, by choosing home birth, to engender a family-oriented closeness. Older siblings can easily be included in an experience normally denied them. . . . Martha could touch our babies immediately. . . . Bill was able to hold our sons even before they were dressed. Martha nursed right away. This cements the mother-child bond (Longbrake and Longbrake, 1979:158–59).

While opponents of home birth believe it to be unconscionably dangerous, its advocates contend that routine active medical management creates a spiraling sequence of interventions:

> Most of the apparent need for hospitalization in birth is created by the hospital itself and the greatest cause for needing obstetrical intervention is obstetricians. By use of IV's and oxytocin [a drug for inducing and augmenting labor] they create fetal distress; they then intervene. By use of fetal monitors and lack of skill in handling breech presentations, they set up a crisis calling for cesarean surgery; they then do the surgery. By polluting the maternal blood stream with analgesic and anesthetic drugs and by impatience in third stage, they cause hemorrhages; they have a ready blood bank to take care of it. By inducing labors by chemicals or breaking the bag of waters, they increase the incidence of prematurity and respiratory distress syndrome in newborns; they have a neonatologist and an intensive care unit to handle it. By frequent, unnecessary internal exams in

labor, by use of internal fetal monitors, and because hospitals house concentrations of harmful germs not found anywhere except in hospitals, they cause infections in both mother and baby; they have the antibiotics to attack it. And so on (Stewart and Stewart, 1979:2).

To these individuals, home birth seems the safer as well as the more humane option.

Physicians' vehement opposition to home births makes it a difficult choice at best. Few are willing to attend home births or provide medical backup for other physicians or nurse-midwives who do. The reemergence of lay midwifery in the United States, the subject of the remainder of this book, stems directly from the difficulties consumers encounter when seeking a trained home birth attendant.

THE WIDER HEALTH CONSUMER MOVEMENT

Parturient women have not been alone in challenging medical ideas, practices, and control. A symbiotic relationship connects the childbirth consumer movement to the holistic and feminist health movements. The latter provide the broader context and philosophy which underpin the childbirth movement, while childbirth has provided critical examples from which alternative philosophy and politics have developed.

Since the late 1960s, feminists have developed both a radical critique of the medical care system and alternatives to that system. Feminists have been prominent critics of medicalization. Childbirth is only one example of the redefinition of women's experiences as medical problems requiring medical solutions. Menstruation, menopause, and aging have met similar fates (for example, McCrea, 1983), and women who do not fit or are unhappy in their assigned gender role are frequently labeled mentally ill by physicians (Brodsky and Hare-Mustin, 1980; Carmen et al., 1981).

The feminist health movement also has pointed to the dangers that arise when higher status individuals control the health care of subordinates (for example, Corea, 1985; Scully, 1977). As researchers have documented, physicians have perpetuated medicine as an upper-class white male enclave (Lorber, 1984; Morantz-Sanchez, 1985; Walsh, 1977). As a result, "the relationship between a woman and her doctor is usually one of profound inequality on every level, an exaggeration of the power imbalance inherent in almost all male-female relationships in our society" (Boston Women's Health Book Collective, 1984:561–62). In these circumstances, clients' needs may be overlooked, their opinions ignored, and the information they provide disbelieved (for example, Armitage et al., 1979; Bernstein and Kane, 1981).

This analysis underpins the alternative services which feminist groups have founded. Organizations such as the Emma Goldman Women's Health Center in Chicago and the Feminist Women's Health Center in Los Angeles differ from traditional health care services in stressing health education and prevention, relying heavily on paramedical workers and lay counselors, and struggling to flatten the hierarchy which generally characterizes health care provision. Feminists also have been active in organizing self-help groups and writing self-help manuals to assist women in maintaining or improving their health, while demystifying medical knowledge and encouraging women to control their own health care. Among the more notable examples are *How to Stay Out of the Gynecologist's Office*, a self-help gynecology textbook (Federation of Feminist Women's Health Centers, 1981); *When Birth Control Fails . . .* , a self-abortion guide (Gage, 1979); and the highly popular *Our Bodies, Ourselves* (Boston Women's Health Collective, 1984), now published in 13 languages.

Although the feminist health movement has provided a radical critique of our health care system, it has not rejected Western medicine or science per se. In contrast, the holistic health movement, begun during the 1970s, presents a more fundamental challenge to American medical philosophies.

The holistic health movement consists of both a philosophy of health care and a broad set of "alternative" healing modalities, such as acupuncture, massage, and yoga. Medical norms envision the human body as a machine and dictate that treatment be restricted to the particular malfunctioning part. Holistic healers reject this mechanistic, reductionist conception of health and illness as limited, ineffective, and dehumanizing. Instead, they believe that health and illness derive from a complex interweaving of psychological, physical, social, and spiritual factors. They attempt to rely on the body's natural healing abilities and encourage clients to find healing power within themselves. Like feminists, they argue that "the healer is merely a facilitator of the healing processes. . . . The healing team does not make the person well, but helps the person to make himself or herself well" (Otto and Knight, 1979:9).

The potential implications of the childbirth consumer movement share similarities with its holistic and feminist counterparts. The childbirth consumer movement, like the holistic movement, must confront the dilemma caused by its focus on personal responsibility. Giving consumers responsibility for their own health care can be an empowering experience, and an effective way to reduce individuals' sense of alienation from their bodies and the health care system. Less motivated or less educated individuals, however, may lack the skills and resources needed to maintain their own health. Yet some holistic practitioners have refused to acknowledge and accept their additional responsibilities with such individuals or have refused to provide services to them. As a result, the quality of care provided may suffer and alternative options may be restricted to better educated, more motivated individuals. At the same time, the emphasis on individual responsibility may decrease awareness of how social, political, and true biological factors can affect health and illness (Crawford, 1979). This can occur when practitioners believe that individuals choose illness as a way of meeting other needs in their lives. The implications for action are quite different if we believe, for example, that cancer is caused by individual desire for attention rather than by industrial pollutants, a viral organism, or internal biological processes. In the extreme, the holistic promotion of individual responsibility unwittingly may foster conservative social trends or keep people from obtaining needed and timely medical intervention.

The feminist health movement may be criticized for providing palliatives that make women's lives more tolerable but do not challenge the basis of patriarchy and sexism. Similarly, the childbirth consumer movement has worked largely to ameliorate the system rather than to change it radically. Certainly it has made the hospital childbirth experience more pleasant for many individual families by winning entry for fathers into labor and delivery rooms and changing medical attitudes about strapping women down and breastfeeding. By doing so, however, it has relieved much consumer dissatisfaction which might otherwise have produced more fundamental structural changes. Those few consumers who refuse to be satisfied with the changes physicians have allowed largely have opted out of the system altogether by choosing home birth. Whereas these individuals may philosophically and psychologically threaten medical perspectives and power, the specter of thousands of families demanding a different kind of care from physicians within hospitals would pose a far greater challenge.

REFERENCES

Ahn, Chung H., and William C. MacLean. "Growth of the exclusively breast-fed infant." *American Journal of Clinical Nutrition* 33:183–92, 1980.

Aldrich, C. Anderson. "The advisability of breastfeeding." *Journal of American Medical Association* 135:915–16, 1947.

Alexander, Shana. "How to make a baby smile: F. Leboyer's revolutionary new approach to childbirth." *Newsweek* 85:84, March 31, 1975.

American Academy of Pediatrics and the American College of Obstetrics and Gynecology. *Guidelines for Perinatal Care.* 1983.

Anderson, G. V. "What kind of anesthetic for childbirth?" excerpt. *Redbook* 124:32+, March 1965.

Anderson, Sandra, Eleanor Bauwens, and Elizabeth Warner. "The choice of home birth in a metropolitan county in Arizona." *Journal of Obstetrics and Gynecological Nursing* 7:41–46, 1978.

Armitage, Karen J., Lawrence J. Schneiderman, and Robert A. Bass. "Response of physicians to medical complaints in men and women." *Journal of the American Medical Association* 241:2186–87, 1979.

Arms, Suzanne. "How hospitals complicate childbirth." *Ms.* 3:108–15, May 1975[a].

Arms, Suzanne. *Immaculate Deception: A New Look at Women and Childbirth in America.* Boston: Houghton Mifflin, 1975[b].

Arney, William R. *Power and the Profession of Obstetrics.* Chicago: University of Chicago Press, 1982.

Atkinson, Stephanie A., Ingeborg C. Radde, and G. Harvey Anderson. "Macromineral balances in premature infants fed their own mothers' milk or formula." *Journal of Pediatrics* 102:99–106, 1983.

Baker, Gretta. "Breast or bottle?" *Redbook* 121:28, August 1963.

Banta, David, and Stephen Thacker. "Electronic fetal monitoring: Is it of benefit?" *Birth and the Family Journal* 6:237–49, 1979.

Banta, David, and Stephen Thacker. "The risks and benefits of episiotomies: A review." *Birth* 9:25–30, 1982.

Baumgarten, K. "Advantages and disadvantages of low amniotomy." *Journal of Perinatal Medicine* 4:3–11, 1976.

Beck, Niels. "Natural childbirth: A review and analysis." *Obstetrics and Gynecology* 52:371–79, 1978.

Beerens, Henri, C. Romond, and C. Neut. "Influence of breast-feeding on the bifid flora of the newborn intestine." *American Journal of Clinical Nutrition* 33:2434–39, 1980.

Bernstein, Barbara, and Robert Kane. "Physicians' attitudes toward female patients." *Medical Care* 19:600–08, 1981.

Bing, Elizabeth. "Childbirth: Liberated labor." *Harper's Bazaar* 110:103+, November 1976.

Blacow, M., M. N. Smith, M. Graham, and R. G. Wilson. "Induction of labour." *Lancet* 1:217, 1975.

Blaikley, John B. "A discussion of the proper place of surgical induction with a review of its hazards." *American Journal of Obstetrics and Gynecology* 71:291–99, 1956.

Borch-Johnsen, K., T. Mandrup-Poulsen, B. Zachau-Christiansen, Geir Jones, M. Christy, K. Kastrup, and J. Nerup. "Relation between breast-feeding and incidence rates of insulin-dependent diabetes mellitus." *Lancet* 2:1083–87, 1984.

Boston Women's Health Book Collective. *The New Our Bodies, Ourselves*. New York: Simon & Schuster, 1984.

Brazelton, T. "What childbirth drugs can do to your child." *Redbook*, 136–65+, February 1971.

Brenner, Patricia, and Robert Brenner. "What really happens when your obstetrician is late." *Ladies Home Journal* 83:42+, June 1966.

British Medical Journal. "Active management of labour." 4:126–27, 1972.

British Medical Journal. "Induction of labour." 3:176–77, 1970.

Brodsky, Annette M., and Rachel Hare-Mustin (eds.). *Women and Psychotherapy: An Assessment of Research and Practices*. New York: Guilford Press, 1980.

Brody, Jane. "Childbirth drugs and your baby." *Redbook* 145:82–3+, August 1975.

Bullen, Catherine L., and A. T. Willis. "Resistance of the breast-fed infant to gastroenteritis." *British Medical Journal* 3:338–43, 1971.

Burnett, Claude A., James A. Jones, Judith Rooks, Chong H. Chen, Carl W. Tyler, and C. Anderson Miller. "Home delivery and neonatal mortality in North Carolina. *Journal of the American Medical Association* 244:2741–45, 1980.

Byers, Tim, Saxon Graham, Thomas Rzepka, and James Marshall. "Lacta-

tion and breast cancer: Evidence for a negative association in premeno-
pausal women." *American Journal of Epidemiology* 121:664–74, 1985.

Caldeyro-Barcia, Roberto. "Some consequences of obstetrical interference."
Birth and the Family Journal 2:34–38, 1975.

Caldeyro-Barcia, Roberto. "Supine called worst position during labor and
delivery." *Obstetrics and Gynecology News*, June:1+, 1975.

Cameron, Joyce, Eileen S. Chase, and Sally O'Neal. "Home birth in Salt Lake
County, Utah." *American Journal of Public Health* 69:716–17, 1979.

Carlson, Regina. "Why nursing a baby means love to me." *Redbook* 142:59+,
December 1973.

Carmen, Elaine (Hilberman), Nancy F. Russo, and Jean B. Miller. "Inequality
and women's mental health: An overview." *American Journal of Psychiatry*
138:1319–30, 1981.

Carro, Geraldine. "Is it safe to breast feed?" *Ladies Home Journal* 95:32+,
March 1978.

Carroll, Gladys H. "I nursed my babies." *Ladies' Home Journal* 64:162–63,
January 1947.

Casey, Clare E., Phillip A. Walravens, and K. Michael Hambidge. "Availability of zinc: Loading tests with human milk, cow's milk and infant formulas."
Pediatrics 68:394–96, 1981.

Casselberry, Ellen. "Forum on malpractice issues in childbirth." *Public Health
Reports* 100:629–33, 1985.

Cave, Carolyn. "Social characteristics of natural childbirth users and non-
users." *American Journal of Public Health* 68:898–901, 1978.

Chalmers, Iain, H. Campbell, and A. C. Turnbull. "Use of oxytocin and
incidence of neonatal jaundice." *British Medical Journal* 2:116–18, 1975.

Chalmers, Iain, M. E. Dauncey, E. R. Verrier-Jones, J. A. Dodge, and O. P.
Gray. "Respiratory distress syndrome in infants of Cardiff residents during 1965–75." *British Medical Journal* 2:1119–21, 1978.

Chew, W. C.. and I. L. Swann. "Influence of simultaneous low amniotomy
and oxytocin infusion and other maternal factors on neonatal jaundice: A
prospective study." *British Medical Journal* 1:72–73, 1977.

Claman, Paul, R. J. Carpenter, and Alex Reiter. "Uterine rupture with the
use of vaginal prostaglandin E$_2$ for induction of labor." *American Journal of
Obstetrics and Gynecology* 150:889–91, 1984.

Clark, Matt. "Back to the breast." *Newsweek* 92:92, November 6, 1978.

Clark, N. "Traditional alternative: Lamaze method at maternity wing of New
York Hospital-Cornell Medical Center." *Harper's Bazaar* 110:103+,
November 1976.

Clinch, J. "Induction of labour: A six year review." *British Journal of Obstetrics
and Gynecology* 86:340–42, 1979.

Cohen, Richard L. "A comparative study of women choosing two different childbirth alternatives." *Birth* 9:13–19, 1982.

Cohen, Nancy W., and Lois J. Estner. *The Silent Knife: Cesarean Prevention and Vaginal Birth after Cesarean.* S. Hadley, MA: Bergin and Garvey, 1983.

Cole, R. A., P. W. Howie, and M. C. Macnaughton. "Elective induction of labour: A randomised prospective trial." *Lancet* 1:767–70, 1975.

Committee on Drugs, American Academy of Pediatrics. "Effect of medication during labor and delivery on infant outcome." *Pediatrics* 62:402–03, 1978.

Committee on Maternal Nutrition, National Academy of Sciences. *Maternal Nutrition and Course of Pregnancy, Summary Report.* Rockville, MD: U.S. Department of Health, Education and Welfare, 1970.

Consumer Reports. "Is breast-feeding best for babies?" 142:152+, March 1977.

Corea, Gena. *The Hidden Malpractice: How American Medicine Mistreats Women.* New York: Harper, 1985.

Cranch, Gene S. "Breast feeding is beautiful." *Parents* 52:50+, October 1977.

Crawford, Robert. "Individual responsibility and health politics," pp. 247–68 in Susan Reverby and David Rosner (eds.), *Health Care in America: Essays in Social History.* Philadelphia: Temple University Press, 1979.

Cunningham, Allan S. "Morbidity in breast-fed and artificially-fed infants." *Journal of Pediatrics* 90:726–29, 1977.

Cunningham, Allan S. "Morbidity in breast-fed and artificially-fed infants II." *Journal of Pediatrics* 95:685–89, 1979.

D'Souza, S. W., T. Macfarlane, and B. Richards. "Effects of oxytocin in induction of labour on neonatal jaundice." *British Journal of Obstetrics and Gynecology* 86:133–38, 1979.

Davidson, B. "Case for and against induced labor." *Good Housekeeping* 158:58–59+, January 1964.

Davis, Elizabeth. *A Guide to Midwifery: Heart and Hands.* Santa Fe: John Muir, 1982.

de Chateau, Peter. "The importance of the neonatal period for the development of synchrony in the mother-infant dyad: A review." *Birth and the Family Journal* 4:10–22, 1977.

De Lee, Joseph B. "The prophylactic forceps operation." *American Journal of Obstetrics and Gynecology* 1:39–40, 1920.

Devitt, Neal. "The transition from home to hospital birth in the United States, 1930–1960." *Birth and the Family Journal* 4:47–58, 1977.

Dick-Read, Grantly. *Natural Childbirth.* London: Heinemann, 1933.

Dick-Read, Grantly. *Childbirth without Fear: The Principles and Practice of Natural Childbirth.* New York: Harper & Brothers, 1944.

Dick-Read, Grantly. "Childbirth without fear and without pain." *Ladies Home Journal* 74:72–73+, June 1957.

Dicker, Richard C., Mark Scully, Joel Greenspan, Peter Layde, Howard Ory, Joyce Maze, and Jack Smith. "Hysterectomy among women of reproductive age." *Journal of the American Medical Association* 248:323–27, 1982.

Dingley, Erma. "Birthplace alternatives." *Oregon Health Bulletin* 55:1–4, 1977.

Dingley, Erma. "Birthplace and attendants: Oregon's alternative experience." *Women and Health* 4:239–53, 1979.

Downham, M. A. P. S., R. Scott, D. G. Sims, J. K. G. Webb, and P. S. Gardner. "Breast-feeding protects against respiratory syncytial virus infections." *British Medical Journal* 2:274–76, 1976.

Dreifus, Claudia (ed.). *Seizing Our Bodies: The Politics of Women's Health.* New York: Vintage, 1977.

Eakins, Pamela S. "Rise of the free-standing birth center: Principles and practice." *Women and Health* 9:49–64, 1984.

Elkins, Valmai H. *The Rights of Pregnant Parents.* New York: Two Continents, 1976.

Ellestad-Sayed, Judith, F. J. Coodin, Louise A. Dilling, and J. C. Haworth. "Breast-feeding protects against infection in Indian infants." *Canadian Medical Association Journal* 120:295–98, 1979.

Erving, H. W., and Anthony N. Kenwick. "Elective induction of labor." *American Journal of Obstetrics and Gynecology* 64:1125–30, 1952.

Fallot, Mary, John L. Boyd, and Frank A. Oski. "Breast-feeding reduces incidences of hospital admissions for infection in infants." *Pediatrics* 65:1121–24, 1980.

Federation of Feminist Women's Health Centers. *How to Stay Out of The Gynecologist's Office.* Los Angeles: Women to Women Publications, 1981.

Feinbloom, Richard. "Natural Childbirth." *Redbook* 142:48+, December 1973.

Fielding, Waldo, and Lois Benjamin. *The Childbirth Challenge: Commonsense Versus "Natural" Methods.* New York: Viking, 1962[a].

Fielding, Waldo, and Lois Benjamin. "Medical case against natural childbirth." *McCalls* 89:106–07, June 1962[b].

Fields, Harry. "Complications of elective induction." *Obstetrics and Gynecology* 15:476–80, 1960.

Forman, M. R., B. I. Graubard, H. J. Hoffman, R. Beren, E. E. Harley, and P. Bennett. "The Pima infant feeding study: Breastfeeding and respiratory infections during the first year of life." *International Journal of Epidemiology* 13:447–53, 1984.

Fraiberg, Selma. *Every Child's Birthright: In Defense of Mothering.* New York: Basic Books, 1977.

France, Gene L., David Marmer, and Russell W. Steele. "Breast feeding and salmonella infection." *American Journal of Diseases of Children* 134:147–52, 1980.

Gage, Suzann. *When Birth Control Fails . . . .* Hollywood: Speculum Press, 1979.

Gaskin, Ina May. *Spiritual Midwifery.* Summertown, TN: The Book Publishing Co., 1975.

Gerbie, Albert. "What happens during labor?" *Redbook* 129:33–34, May 1967.

Gerrard, John W. "Breast-feeding: Second thoughts." *Pediatrics* 54:757–64, 1974.

Goldfarb, Johanna, and Edith Tibbetts. *Breastfeeding Handbook.* Hillside, NJ: Enslow, 1980.

Goldfarb, M., and R. Goldfarb. "We shared our baby's birth." *Ladies Home Journal* 75:140+, December 1958.

Good Housekeeping. "Childbirth: When labor is induced." 153:147, September 1961.

Good Housekeeping. "Why forceps may be used in delivering a baby." 161:145, August 1965.

Good Housekeeping. "Why women may fail in breast feeding." 157:140, August 1963.

Gorbach, Arthur. "What to expect during labor and delivery." *Redbook* 140:65+, December 1972.

Grace of Monaco. "Why mothers should breast-feed their babies." *Ladies Home Journal* 88:56+, August 1971.

Gross, Steven J., and Edda Gabriel. "Vitamin E status in preterm infants fed human milk or infant formula." *Journal of Pediatrics* 106:635–39, 1985.

Grossman, M. "Natural childbirth was easy for me." *Parents Magazine* 34:36–37, January 1959.

Gurney, William. "Natural childbirth comes of age." *Reader's Digest* 103:153–56, December 1973.

Gyorgy, Paul, Sakhorn Dhanamitta, and Edward Steers. "Protective effects of human milk in experimental staphylococcal infections." *Science* 137:338–39, 1962.

Haire, Doris. *The Cultural Warping of Childbirth.* Seattle: International Childbirth Education Association, 1972.

Harris, Julie. "I was afraid to have a baby." *McCalls* 84:68+, December 1956.

Haynes de Regt, Roberta, Howard L. Minkoff, Joseph Feldman, and Richard

H. Schwartz. "Relation of private or clinic care to the cesarean birth rate." *New England Journal of Medicine* 315:619–24, 1986.

Hazell, Lester D. *Birth Goes Home.* Seattle: Catalyst Publishing, 1974.

Hazell, Lester D. "A study of 300 elective home births." *Birth and the Family Journal* 2:11–18, 1975.

Henig, Robin M. "The case for mother's milk." *New York Times Sunday Magazine,* 40+, July 8, 1979.

Hide, D. W., and B. M. Guyer. "Clinical manifestations of allergy related to breast- and cow's milk-feeding." *Pediatrics* 76:972–75, 1985.

Hoover, M. "Hidden rewards of childbirth training." *McCalls* 101:59, February 1974.

Hoyle, Bruce, M. Yunus, and Lincoln C. Chen. "Breast feeding and food intake among children with acute diarrheal diseases." *American Journal of Clinical Nutrition* 33:2365–71, 1980.

Hughes, R. N., and J. A. Bushnell. "Further relationships between IPAT anxiety scale performance and infantile feeding experiences." *Journal of Clinical Psychology* 33:698–700, 1977.

Hughes, R. N, and Anthea B. Hawkins. "EPI and IPAT anxiety scale performance in young women as related to breast feeding during infancy." *Journal of Clinical Psychology* 31:663–65, 1975.

Hughey, Michael, Thomas McElin, and Todd Young. "Maternal and fetal outcomes of Lamaze-prepared patients." *Obstetrics and Gynecology* 51:643–47, 1978.

Husbands, Tom L. "Elective induction of labor." *American Journal of Obstetrics and Gynecology* 60:900–03, 1950.

Ing, Roy, J. H. C. Ho, and Nicholas L. Petrakis. "Unilateral breast-feeding and breast cancer." *Lancet* 2:124–27, 1977.

Ingemarsson, E., I. Ingemarsson, and M. Westgren. "Combined decelerations—clinical significance and relationship to uterine activity." *Obstetrics and Gynecology* 58:35, 1981.

Interprofessional Task Force on Health Care in Women and Children. *Joint Position Statement on the Development of Family-Centered Maternity/Newborn Care in Hospitals.* Washington, DC: American College of Obstetricians and Gynecologists, 1978.

Janas, Lynn M., Mary F. Pecciano, and Terry Hatch. "Indices of protein metabolism in term infants fed human milk, whey-predominant formula, or cow's milk formula." *Pediatrics* 75:775–84, 1985.

Kalkstein, S. "Miracle of the beginning: A child is born." *Good Housekeeping* 172:62–65, January 1971.

Karmel, Marjorie. *Thank You, Dr. Lamaze: A Mother's Experience in Painless Childbirth.* New York: Doubleday, 1959.

Kenyon, Josephine H. "The breast-fed baby." *Good Housekeeping* 123:78+, September 1946.

Klaus, Marshall H., and John H. Kennell. *Maternal-Infant Bonding*. St. Louis: C. V. Mosby, 1976.

Koepsell, T. D., N. Weiss, D. Thompson, and D. Martin. "Prevalence of prior hysterectomy in the Seattle-Tacoma area." *American Journal of Public Health* 70:40–47, 1980.

Koop, C. Everett, and M. Elizabeth Brannon. "Breast feeding—the community norm. Report of a workshop." *Public Health Reports* 99:550–58, 1984.

Kramer, Michael S. "Do breast-feeding and delayed introduction of solid foods protect against subsequent obesity?" *Journal of Pediatrics* 98:883–87, 1981.

Kramer, Michael S., Ronald G. Barr, Denis G. Leduc, Christiane Boijoly, Lynn McVey-White, and Barry Pless. "Determinants of weight and adiposity in the first year of life." *Journal of Pediatrics* 106:10–14, 1985.

Ladies Home Journal. "Natural Childbirth: Facts and Fallacies." 79:53+, October 1962.

Ladies Home Journal. "Is the breast best?" 92:24, October 1975.

Lake, Alice. "Childbirth in America." *McCalls* 103:83+, January 1976.

La Leche League International. *The Womanly Art of Breastfeeding*. Franklin Park, IL, 1958.

Lamaze, Fernand. *Painless Childbirth*. London: Burke, 1958.

Lancet. "Induction of labour for postmaturity." 1:1225, 1982.

Lancet. "A time to be born." 2:1183–84, 1974.

Lang, Raven. *The Birth Book*. Palo Alto, CA: Genesis, 1972.

Larsen, Spencer A., and Daryl R. Homer. "Relation of breast vs. bottle feeding to hospitalization for gastroenteritis in a middle class U.S. population." *Journal of Pediatrics* 92:417–18, 1978.

Lehrer, Steven. "Breastfeeding and immunity." *Harpers* 108:50+, July 1975.

Lepage, Phillippe, Christophe Munyakazi, and Phillippe Hennart. "Breast-feeding and hospital mortality in children in Rwanda." *Lancet* 2:409–11, 1981.

Lesko, Wendy. "The birth chart." *Good Housekeeping* 202:123–26, June 1986.

Leveno, Kenneth J., F. Gary Cunningham, Sheryl Nelson, Micki Rourk, M. Lynne Williams, David Guzick, Sharon Dowling, Charles R. Rosenfeld, and Ann Buckley. "A prospective comparison of selective and universal electronic fetal monitoring in 34,995 pregnancies." *New England Journal of Medicine* 315:615–18, 1986.

Liston, W. A., and A. J. Campbell. "Dangers of oxytocin-induced labour to fetuses." *British Medical Journal* 3:606–07, 1974.

Longbrake, Martha, and William A. Longbrake. "Control is the key," pp.

154–59 in David Stewart and Lee Stewart (eds.), *Compulsory Hospitalization or Freedom of Choice in Childbirth*, Vol. 1. Marble Hill, MO: NAPSAC Reproductions, 1979.

Longwell, M. "Happiest way to have a baby: St. Mary's hospital, Evansville, Ind., family centered maternity care unit." *Farm Journal* 90:84–85+, 1966.

Lorber, Judith. *Women Physicians: Careers, Status and Power*. New York: Tavistock, 1984.

Lubin, A. H., R. O. Shrock, and J. L. Bonner. "Iron status of breast-fed and formula-fed infants at age 6 months." *Journal of Pediatrics* 98:1019–20, 1981.

Lynaugh, Kathleen H. "The effects of early elective amniotomy on the length of labor and the condition of the fetus." *Journal of Nurse-Midwifery* 25:3–9, 1980.

MacDonald, Dermot. "Surgical induction of labor." *American Journal of Obstetrics and Gynecology* 107:908–11, 1970.

Maisels, M. Jeffrey, Richard Rees, Keith Marks, and Zev Freidman. "Elective delivery of the term fetus: An obstetrical hazard." *Journal of the American Medical Association* 238:2036–39, 1977.

Marshall, M. "My husband delivered our baby." *Good Housekeeping* 179:77–78+, September 1974.

Martin, D. H., W. Thompson, J. H. M. Pinkerton, and J. D. Watson. "A randomised controlled trial of selective planned delivery." *British Journal of Obstetrics and Gynecology* 85:109–13, 1978.

Martinez, G. A., D. Dodd, and J. Samartgedes. "Milk feeding patterns in the U.S. during the first twelve months of life," unpublished paper. Ross Laboratories, March 6, 1981.

McCalls. "Doctor talks about babies by appointment." 84:4+, January 1957.

McCrea, Frances. "The politics of menopause." *Social Problems* 31:111–23, 1983.

McNay, Margaret B., Gillian M. McIlwaine, P. W. Howie, and M. C. MacNaughton. "Perinatal deaths: Analysis by clinical cause to assess value of induction of labour." *British Medical Journal* 1:347–50, 1977.

Mehl, Lewis, and Gail H. Peterson. "Home birth versus hospital birth." Paper presented at the meeting of the American Public Health Association, Miami, Florida, October 20, 1976.

Mendels, Ora. "Revolution in childbirth?" *Ladies Home Journal* 80:40, January 1963.

Meyer, H. F. "Breastfeeding in the United States: Extent and possible trend." *Pediatrics* 22:116–21, 1958.

Miles, Lee M. "Elective induction of labor at term." *American Journal of Obstetrics and Gynecology* 62:649–53, 1951.

Milinaire, C. "Born happy." *Vogue* 164:80–81+, July 1974.

Miller, H. Lloyd, Francis E. Flannery, and Dorothy Bell. "Education for childbirth in private practice: 450 consecutive cases." *American Journal of Obstetrics and Gynecology* 63:792–99, 1952.

Moran, James D., and Nancy von Bargen. "Attitudinal and demographic factors influencing mother's choice of childbirth procedures." *American Journal of Obstetrics and Gynecology* 142:846–50, 1982.

Morantz-Sanchez, Regina M. *Sympathy and Science: Women Physicians in American Medicine.* New York: Oxford University Press, 1985.

Murray, A. B. "Infant feeding and respiratory allergy." *Lancet* 1:497, 1971.

Myers, Martin G., Samuel J. Fomon, Franklin P. Koonty, Gail A. McGuinness, Peter A. Lachenbruch, and Rachel Hollingshead. "Respiratory and gastrointestinal illnesses in breast- and formula-fed infants." *American Journal of Diseases of Children* 138:629–32, 1984.

Narayanan, Indira, Shashi Bala, K. Prakash, R. K. Verma, and V. V. Gujral. "Partial supplementation with expressed breast-milk for prevention of infection in low-birth-weight infants." *Lancet* 2:561–63, 1980.

Narayanan, Indira, K. Prakash, and V. V. Gujral. "The value of human milk in the prevention of infection in the high-risk low-birth-weight infant." *Journal of Pediatrics* 99:496–98, 1981.

Narayanan, Indira, N. S. Murthy, K. Prakash, and V. V. Gujral. "Randomised controlled trial of effect of raw and holder pasteurized human milk and of formula supplements on incidence of neonatal infection." *Lancet* 2:1111–13, 1984.

National Center for Health Statistics. "Advance report of final natality statistics, 1984." *Monthly Vital Statistics Report* 35 (4) supplement, 1986.

National Center for Health Statistics. S. Taffel. "Maternal weight gain and the outcome of pregnancy, United States, 1980." *Vital and Health Statistics Series* 21, no. 44, DHHS Publication No. 86-1922, Public Health Service. Washington, DC: U.S. Government Printing Office, June 1986.

Newsweek. "Natural or unnatural?" 65:97, March 15, 1965

Newsweek. "Return to breast-feeding?" 75:62–63, January 12, 1970[a].

Newsweek. "Birth by appointment." 76:85, July 20, 1970[b].

NICHD National Registry for Amniocentesis Study Group. "Midtrimester amniocentesis for prenatal diagnosis: Safety and accuracy." *Journal of the American Medical Association* 236: 1471–76, 1976.

Nolen, W. "Induced labor: When is it a good idea?" *McCalls* 98:24–51, July 1971.

Nutrition Committee of the Canadian Paediatric Society and the Committee on Nutrition of the American Academy of Pediatrics. "Breast feeding: A commentary in celebration of the International Year of the Child, 1979." *Pediatrics* 62:591–601, 1978.

Oberkotter, Linda V., Gilberto R. Pereira, Mary H. Paul, Henry Ling, Sharon Sasanow, and Martin Farber. "Effect of breast-feeding vs. formula-feeding on circulating thyroxine levels in premature infants." *Journal of Pediatrics* 106:822–25, 1985.

O'Driscoll, Kieran, Reginald J. Jackson, and John T. Gallagher. "Prevention of prolonged labour." *British Medical Journal* 2:477–80, 1969.

O'Driscoll, Kieran, John M. Stronge, and Maurice Minogue. "Active management of labour." *British Medical Journal* 3:135–37, 1973.

O'Keefe, Margaret. "We're twenty years behind in breast feeding." *Ladies Home Journal* 79:70+, November 1962.

O'Leary, James L., and James A. O'Leary. "The complete episiotomy." *Obstetrics and Gynecology* 25:235–40, 1965.

Ostapowicz, F. "Anesthesia and analgesia during childbirth." *Redbook* 136:12+, April 1971.

Otto, Herbert A., and James W. Knight. "Wholistic healing: Basic principles and concepts," pp. 3–27 in Herbert A. Otto and James W. Knight (eds.), *Dimensions in Wholistic Healing: New Frontiers in the Treatment of the Whole Person*. Chicago: Nelson-Hall, 1979.

Palkovitz, Rob. "Fathers' birth attendance, early extended contact, and father-infant interaction at five months postpartum." *Birth* 9:173–77, 1982.

Parents Magazine. "Breast or bottle for a baby?" 20:20+, August 1945.

Parents Magazine. "They wanted to nurse their babies." 25:36+, October 1950.

Parents Magazine. "Natural childbirth: Lamaze Method." 46:56–59, March 1971.

Pearce, J. M. F., J. H. Sheperd, and C. D. Sims. "Prostaglandin E_2 pessaries for induction of labour." *Lancet* 1:572–75, 1979.

Pearse, Warren H. "To section or not to section." *American Journal of Public Health* 73:843–44, 1983.

Persico, M., L. Podoskin, M. Frades, D. Golan, and G. Wellisch. "Recurrent middle ear infections in infants: Protective role of maternal breast-feeding." *Ear, Nose and Throat Journal* 62:20–31, 1983.

Peterson, Gail H., and Lewis E. Mehl. "Parental/child psychology: Delivery alternatives." *Women and Health* 2:3–16, 1977.

Picciano, Mary F., and Ronald H. Deering. "The influence of feeding regimens on iron status during infancy." *American Journal of Clinical Nutrition* 33:746–53, 1980.

Powers, Thomas. "Fathers in the delivery room." *Good Housekeeping* 179:93+, November 1974.

Pryor, Karen. "They teach the joys of breast-feeding." *Readers' Digest* 82:103–06, May 1963.

Rawlins, Carolyn M. "Should you nurse your baby?" *Redbook* 131:44, July 1968.

Reader's Digest. "Doctor talks about babies by appointment." 71:48–50, July 1957.

Reuben, David. "Dr. David Reuben answers your questions about breast feeding." *McCalls* 98:64+, May 1971.

Reycraft, James L. "Induction of labor." *American Journal of Obstetrics and Gynecology* 61:801–05, 1951.

Riker, Audrey P. "Nursing comes naturally." *Parents* 35:38+, February 1960.

Roberts, Joyce. "Alternative positions for childbirth. Part 1: First stage of labor." *Journal of Nurse-Midwifery* 25:11–20, 1980a.

Roberts, Joyce. "Alternative positions for childbirth. Part 2: Second stage of labor." *Journal of Nurse-Midwifery* 25:13–20, 1980b.

Rothman, Barbara Katz. "Awake and aware, or false consciousness: The cooption of childbirth reform in America," pp. 150–80 in Shelly Romalis (ed.), *Childbirth: Alternatives to Medical Control.* Austin: University of Texas Press, 1981.

Saarinen, Ulla M., Alf Bachman, Merja Kajosaari, and Martti Siimes. "Prolonged breast-feeding as prophylaxis for atopic disease." *Lancet* 2:163–66, 1979.

Sandelowski, Margarete. *Pain, Pleasure, and American Childbirth: From the Twilight Sleep to the Read Method, 1914–1960.* Westport, CT: Greenwood Press, 1984.

Saturday Evening Post. "Breast milk is best." 251:107, April 1979.

Schreiner, S. "Toward a new way to birth: Theories of F. Leboyer." *Reader's Digest* 108:140–43, January 1976.

Scully, Diana. *Men who Control Women's Health: The Miseducation of Obstetrician-Gynecologists.* Boston: Houghton Mifflin, 1980.

Searles, Carolyn. "The impetus toward home birth." *Journal of Nurse-Midwifery* 26:51–56, 1981.

Seligmann, Jean. "New science of birth." *Newsweek* 88:55–56+, November 15, 1976.

Senn, Milton. "Storm over childbirth: The most controversial issue in modern medicine." *McCalls* 9:40+, February 1963.

Sensibar, J. "Why we chose natural childbirth." *Redbook* 132:22+, January 1969.

Shultz, Gladys D. "Breast-feeding miracle." *Ladies Home Journal* 72:93, September 1955.

Shultz, Gladys D. "Journal mothers report on cruelty in maternity wards." *Ladies Home Journal* 75:44–45+, August 1958[a].

Shultz, Gladys D. "Journal mothers testify to cruelty in maternity wards." *Ladies Home Journal*, 75:58–59+, December 1958[b].

Singer, J. E., M. Westphal, and K. Niswander. "Relationship of weight gain during pregnancy to birth weight and infant growth and development in the first year of life." *Obstetrics and Gynecology* 31 (3), March 1968.

Smart, Russell C. "In defense of bottles for babies." *Parents* 35+, April 1950.

Smith, C. P., B. A. Nagourney, F. H. McLean, and R. H. Usher. "Hazards and benefits of elective induction of labor." *American Journal of Obstetrics and Gynecology* 148:579–85, 1984.

Spero, R. "Father watches the birth of his son: Natural childbirth." *Redbook* 125:54–55+, May 1965.

Spock, Benjamin. "How important is breast feeding?" *Ladies Home Journal* 74:26+, March 1957.

Stewart, David, and Lee Stewart. *Compulsory Hospitalization or Freedom of Choice in Childbirth*, Vol. 1. Marble Hill, MO: NAPSAC Reproductions, 1979.

Sullivan, Deborah A., and Ruth Beeman. "Satisfaction with postpartum care: Opportunities for bonding, reconstructing the birth and instruction." *Birth and the Family Journal* 8:153–59, 1981.

Sullivan, Deborah A., and Ruth Beeman. "Satisfaction with maternity care: A matter of communication and choice." *Medical Care* 20:321–30, 1982.

Sumner, Philip E., and Celeste R. Phillips. *Birthing Rooms: Concept and Reality*. St. Louis: C. V. Mosby, 1981.

Sutherland, Donald. "Childbirth is not for mothers only." *Ms.* 2:47–51, May 1974.

Taffel, Selma, Paul Placek, and Mary Moien. "One fifth of U.S. births by cesarean section." *American Journal of Public Health* 75:190, 1985.

Thoms, Herbert, and Robert H. Wyatt. "One thousand consecutive deliveries under a training for childbirth program." *American Journal of Obstetrics and Gynecology* 61:205–09, 1951.

Time. "Fewer drugs for happier mothers." 84:81, September 25, 1964.

Time. "To nurse or not to nurse?" 85:68, April 23, 1965.

Time. "Back to the breast." 92:53–54, July 19, 1968.

Time. "Relieving pressure and pain: Use of decompression unit." 90:36, December 22, 1967.

Torres, T. "From womb to world: A nonviolent transition; the Leboyer method." *Ms.* 3:22, July 1974.

Twenty-seventh World Health Assembly. Part 1: Infant Nutrition and

Breastfeeding. *Official Records of the World Health Organization,* No. 217:20, 1974.

U.S. Bureau of the Census. *Historical Statistics of the United States, Colonial Times to 1970, Bicentennial Edition, Part 1.* Washington, DC: U.S. Government Printing Office, 1975.

U.S. Bureau of the Census. *Statistical Abstracts of the US.: 1985* (105th ed.). Washington, DC: U.S. Government Printing Office, 1984.

U.S. Public Health Service. *Maternity Care Utilization and Financing,* Health Economics Series No. 947-4. Washington, DC: U.S. Government Printing Office, 1964.

U.S. Public Health Service. *Cesarean Childbirth,* NIH Publication No. 82-2967. Washington, DC: U.S. Government Printing Office, 1981.

Walsh, Mary R. *"Doctors Wanted: No Women Need Apply": Sexual Barriers in the Medical Profession, 1835–1975.* New Haven: Yale University Press, 1977.

Warren, Robert J., Martha L. Lepow, Glenn E. Bartsch, and Frederick C. Robbins. "The relationship of maternal antibody, breast-feeding and age to the susceptibility of newborn infants to infection with attenuated polioviruses." *Pediatrics* 34:4–13, 1964.

Weber, Melva. "Baby's plus: Breast feeding." *Vogue* 169:179+, July 1979.

Weitz, Rose, and Deborah Sullivan. "Licensed lay midwifery and the medical model of childbirth." *Sociology of Health and Illness* 7:36–54, 1985.

Wertz, Richard W., and Dorothy C. Wertz. *Lying-In: A History of Childbirth in America.* New York: Free Press, 1977.

Wessel, Morris A. "Breast feeding made easy." *Parents Magazine* 40:70+, November 1965.

Williams, G. "Natural childbirth comes of age." *Reader's Digest* 103:153–56, 1973.

Wilson, J. Robert. "Elective induction of labor: Is it justifiable in normally pregnant women?" *American Journal of Obstetrics and Gynecology* 65:848–54, 1953.

Winberg, J., and George Wessner. "Does breast milk protect against septicaemia in the newborn?" *Lancet* 1:1091–94, 1971.

Woodbury, R. M. "The relation between breast and artificial feeding and infant mortality." *American Journal of Hygiene* 2:668–87, 1922.

World Health Organization. "Appropriate technology for birth." *Lancet* 8452:436–37, 1985.

Wright, Erna. *The New Childbirth.* New York: Hart, 1966.

Wylie, Evan. "I can't believe I'm having a baby!" *Good Housekeeping* 168:72–73, January 1969.

Yoshioka, Hajime, Ken-ichi Iseki, and Kozo Fujita. "Development and differences in intestinal flora in the neonatal period in breast-fed and bottle-fed infants." *Pediatrics* 72:317–21, 1983.

Yudkin, Patricia, A. M. Frumar, Anne B. M. Anderson, and A. C. Turnbull. "A retrospective study of induction of labor." *British Journal of Obstetrics and Gynecology* 86:257–65, 1979.

Yuncker, Barbara. "Baby bubble." *Ladies Home Journal* 86:106–07, September 1969.

Yuncker, Barbara. "Delivery procedures that endanger a baby's life." *Good Housekeeping* 181:56+, August 1975.

CHAPTER 3
THE MIDWIVES

It is difficult to discern a common element in the background of lay midwives. Some come from the affluent homes of doctors, judges, engineers, and corporate executives. Others grew up on farms or in blue collar households. Most of their mothers were housewives but the exceptions ranged from clerical workers to professional career women with doctoral degrees. Many of the midwives have attended college and a small number have master's degrees. Others have only a high school education. Before becoming midwives they worked as housepainters, fashion models, radio broadcasters, secretaries, teachers, chemists, nuns, nurses, and myriad other occupations. Most are married and have children. Their husbands' occupations, like their parents', span a broad range from carpenters and artists to physicians and university professors, and their household incomes vary from under $15,000 to over $50,000. What unites these diverse women is a similar philosophy about health care and a belief that they have been called to provide an alternative to the standard maternity care offered by medical practitioners.

The U.S. data presented in this and subsequent chapters are taken from interviews in 1982 and 1983 with 50 lay midwives in two states—one where lay midwifery is both legal and regulated and one where it is neither regulated nor, at the time of the interviews, legal. In the first state, Arizona, 27 of the 28 women who practiced as licensed midwives at any time between January 1977 and August 1982 were interviewed. The one exception had left the country. In the second state, located in the Northeast, 24 lay midwives working as unsupervised practitioners were identified through international,

national, and state childbirth organizations and snowball sampling; 23 of these were interviewed. The one who declined to be interviewed was involved in a current legal case. There also were reports of a midwife in an isolated religious commune in this state, but not enough information could be obtained to make contact with her.

Interviews were based on a semistructured questionnaire containing open- and close-ended questions about background, training, motivations, attitudes, experiences with medical personnel, and perceptions of obstacles to practice. The interviews averaged about three hours and ranged from two to five hours. All were taped and transcribed.

DEMOGRAPHIC CHARACTERISTICS

Unlike the traditional granny midwives at the turn of the century, all 50 interviewed midwives are white women.[1] A black traditional midwife had practiced in Arizona in the early 1970s before returning to Africa, and there were unconfirmed reports that a black midwife had practiced in the nonregulating state a few years before the study. Since the interviews were conducted, a male midwife has been licensed in Arizona along with 23 additional women. (The large increase resulted from the graduation of two classes from the state-sponsored training program and a one-year grace period that loosened the requirements for licensure.)

The interviewed midwives range in age from the mid-twenties to the early sixties, with the majority in their thirties. Most of those in their thirties have three children compared to the national average of less than two. Only 7 of the 50 had not borne a child at the time of the interview, and most of these intend to have children in the future.

THE PULL OF MIDWIFERY

The virtual eradication of midwifery in the United States has left its mark on the occupational structure. The development of certified

1. Indian Health Service officials in Arizona agree that no Native American midwives practice in the state, since free health care over the last century eliminated their market. According to the Arizona Department of Health Services, no Mexican or Mexican-American licensed midwives have practiced since the 1960s, and unlicensed ones delivery at most a handful of births each year.

nurse-midwives is too recent, and their number too small, for midwifery to be a visible career option for young women. Consequently,
few of the lay midwives considered becoming a midwife until after
their own childbirth experiences. The exceptions include one Por-
tuguese and three British women who grew up in societies where
midwifery is a respectable occupation for a woman, on a par with
teaching. Three others belong to an isolated, traditional, Mormon
community where they provide all primary health care. These three
work in consultation with a few sympathetic outside physicians who
recognize the need for midwives in a remote area where ten or more
children per woman is not uncommon.

Only a small number of the lay midwives from mainstream American backgrounds were interested in maternity care at an early age. In
several cases their interest was linked to an early involvement in
"alternative" lifestyles which stressed self-sufficiency. Half a dozen
others wanted to work in childbirth but had reservations about standard maternity care. The invisibility of midwifery meant that few of
these women knew others who shared their interest or knew how to
obtain training in midwifery. For them, it was a "lone struggle."

In contrast, the majority quickly point out that they did not "actually, consciously decide to become a midwife." Instead, they report
that "it was more of an evolution" or "the path where the river took
me." Some of the midwives had already worked in women's health
care as nurses, childbirth educators, venereal disease screeners, La
Leche advisers, and abortion counselors. During their own pregnancies, they read widely on maternity care. Their reading led to a concern with prevailing maternity care practices and an interest in natural childbirth.

The midwives' own childbirth experiences reinforced their interest in alternative forms of maternity care. In spite of the difficulty
of finding a trained home birth attendant, nearly two-thirds of the
Arizona midwives with children and three-quarters in the northeastern state have had home births. Several others had planned
home births but were transported to a hospital before delivery when
complications arose. The positive aspects of these home birth experiences, even among those who had to be transported, reinforced their
commitment to alternatives in maternity care.

Approximately half the midwives have had a hospital birth. Only a few of these report upsetting personal experiences. One describes the first of her five births 17 years before as a "classical drugged birth, forceps delivery" that put her "in recovery for 24 hours." Another spoke emotionally of a miscalculated preterm induction without her consent, inattentive hospital staff, a poorly healed episiotomy, and a postpartum infection that left her feeling like she "had been raped" and "diminished in terms of being a woman." More frequently the midwives report that their hospital births were "quite normal" but involved "manipulation and control taken away" from them against their wishes. Some say they were frustrated when their physicians, who had agreed to a "natural birth," or the receiving hospital staff ordered medication and fetal monitors, ruptured their membranes, cut episiotomies, and prevented immediate postpartum family bonding. They subsequently began to question whether it was possible to have the kind of childbirth they wanted in a hospital setting.

Even at this point, however, few of the women decided to become midwives. Instead, they tried to find committed physicians who would provide family-centered natural childbirth. One group resorted to soliciting on local television for a physician to attend home births. In the northeastern state, approximately seven physicians have at some time in the last ten years attended planned home births on a regular basis. The number in Arizona was even fewer.

Of the few physicians sympathetic to low intervention, family-centered childbirth, even fewer could devote the time needed to give the personalized care desired, especially for women who wanted home births. As a result, some physicians began using volunteer or paid birth assistants. Two Arizona women and nine northeastern women began their involvement in midwifery in this way. They monitored labors in hospitals or homes, made postpartum visits to homes, and, in some cases, conducted prenatal examinations in the physicians' offices. Their responsibilities grew over time and included delivering home births when the physicians did not arrive in time. A few developed their own clientele of women determined to have a home birth but who could not afford the physicians' fees or lived outside the physicians' practice areas. Later, clients came who felt more comfortable without a physician at their birth. Others developed their own clientele when the physicians with whom they worked ceased attending home births. Four of the seven northeastern physicians, including two family practitioners associated with a medical school, stopped under pressure from colleagues, while another lost his license.

The rest of the women were "backed into midwifery" without having apprenticed with physicians when they perceived a "need" for an alternative. Commonly, these women had their first midwifery experience when a friend decided to give birth at home and could not find a trained attendant. As one of these women explained, "I felt a very, very strong need inside to be responsible, to help her if she had some problems." As an obstetrical nurse, she had seen "a lot of the insults being done to women in the hospital—the manipulation and control taken away. . . . I felt that there had to be something more beautiful, something more unique for each person."

Most of the women did not initially consider themselves midwives. Instead, each generally thought of herself as someone who knew a little more about birth than the average person and was just helping out a friend. They only reluctantly accepted the label and role of midwife when their clients pushed it on them. Some mention that they acknowledged their own identity as midwives only when they first purchased a brass scale or other piece of equipment for their birth kit.

THE STRUGGLE FOR TRAINING

Women who decide to assist at births or become midwives face tremendous difficulties in obtaining training. As discussed in chapters 1 and 2, the slow emergence of national health care regulation in the United States worked against upgrading and institutionalizing midwifery training, so few established means for obtaining such training exist.

Many of the women gained their initial knowledge through consumer study groups. By the early 1970s, growing numbers of women had become concerned about the physical, psychological, and social side effects of standard hospital obstetrics. They joined together in study groups to share information about less interventionist, more family-centered maternity care. Several national organizations formed to assist in establishing and coordinating local groups. The groups range from the relatively conservative International Childbirth Education Association, which promotes psychoprophylactic alternatives to drugs and lobbies for family bonding in hospitals, to the more radical Association for Childbirth at Home and Informed Homebirth, Inc.

Eleven of the 27 Arizona midwives and 19 of the 23 northeastern midwives report attending one of the more radical childbirth study groups. Most went in the hope of finding a physician who shared their reservations about routine medical and surgical intervention in hospital births. In both states, one small group evolved into a structured training program for "birth attendants" to assist self-trained, lay midwives and sympathetic physicians.

The Arizona group became the Arizona School for Midwifery, run by a self-trained lay midwife's husband. He hired foreign-trained midwives and certified nurse-midwives to assist his wife in the coursework. A few physicians gave seminars as well. When Arizona's lay midwifery licensure program was revised and reactivated in 1978, the state recognized completion of the unaccredited program as fulfilling the requirement for formal instruction. Reports from former students who passed the licensure examination, including three who were also registered nurses, indicate an unevenness in the coursework. As a result, they had to do additional study on their own to pass the examination. They also complained that the school did not provide them with the 25 supervised births required by the revised law.

This proprietary school folded in 1981 rife with internal dissension and financial difficulties, leaving students with no way to obtain the training required for licensure. Subsequently, the State Bureau of Maternal and Child Health initiated a three-year demonstration program in midwifery training at a community college in a remote rural area. The program was designed around a series of teaching modules, so it could be adopted by other state colleges. The original program has now ended, and no college has offered the course since. Consequently, the lack of a training program has made the requirement of formal training the catch-22 of the licensure program.

In the northeastern state, an unaccredited, proprietary course run by self-trained midwives also developed in the mid-1970s. It has had greater stability and consistency in quality of training than the Arizona program despite the questionable legal status of lay midwifery there. The basic course now attracts more out-of-state than in-state students. The lay midwife who runs the course is a former chemist married to a university professor. She takes pride in the academic orientation of her course and its reputation as a "very tough course." The course consists of 11 day-long class meetings spread over eight months. A month before each class, students receive an extensive reading list from the standard midwifery and obstetrical textbooks and medical journals. They are expected to know the reading material before coming to class for discussion and demonstration. At the end of each day a test is given and those who do not pass it, or the optional retest, are dropped from the program. On average, only half of the 20 students in the previous eight sessions completed the course successfully. The failure rate has declined in the most recent session, when an excess number of applications resulted in greater selectivity.

Successful completion of the basic course, according to the program brochure, lays the groundwork for becoming a midwife "through apprenticeship with an experienced attendant." An advanced course has now been developed for practicing midwives. At the time of the interviews the course director and several other experienced lay midwives who had been lobbying for the legalization of lay midwifery in their state joined to draw up apprenticeship guidelines and standards for practice as part of a voluntary credential program. They have subsequently become incorporated as a professional trade association. Applicants' experience and training are reviewed by three members with whom she has not worked. At the time of this writing, 20 members have been accepted and approximately 100 applications are pending.

In Arizona, 5 of the 27 licensed midwives were registered nurses at the time of the interviews, including 3 with graduate training in nursing. Another 3 were trained as practical nurses. These 3 and 2 others without formal midwifery training apprenticed with lay midwives before beginning practice. Another 12 received their training through the Arizona School for Midwifery while 2 are British State Certified Midwives.

All the licensed midwives in Arizona have attended workshops sponsored or cosponsored by the Bureau of Maternal and Child Health and conducted by obstetricians, neonatologists, neonatal nurse-practitioners, and pediatricians. In addition, most have attended emergency medical treatment classes, cardiopulmonary resuscitation (CPR) classes, the Arizona Perinatal Trust's continuing education programs, and workshops run by Informed Homebirth and the Association for Childbirth at Home. The midwives have begun to assume some responsibility for their own continuing education and have arranged workshops on resuscitation, pelvic examinations, and physical assessment.

In the northeastern state, with the exception of two foreign-trained midwives, one of whom left the state to go to England for her training, none of the currently practicing midwives came close to meeting the training requirements adopted by the professional trade association before beginning practice. The midwife who teaches the course and eight others, including five registered nurses, began their training in the mid-1970s by working as "birth assistants" to physicians who attended home births. Two of these helped design the basic course, and two have completed it. Some of those who worked with physicians feel that these associations "gradually worked into an apprenticeship without that ever being stated." Others acknowledge that while they viewed their increased responsibility as an apprenticeship, few of the physicians did. Their first deliveries usually occurred when the baby arrived before the physician.

Seven other midwives, including two registered nurses, learned their skills by taking the basic course and then apprenticing with a more experienced lay midwife. Of the remaining five, two worked with other self-trained midwives before beginning their own practices and two were registered nurses who worked in obstetrics. One's only preparation was reading some midwifery and obstetrical textbooks.

Most called themselves "birth attendants" rather than midwives with their early clients, carefully explaining their inexperience and declining monetary compensation. One midwife's own home birth experience illustrates the common level of inexperience; her midwife did not recognize that her baby was posterior (facing the wrong direction) or that she had a second degree laceration. Another, reflecting on her first births, says, "I must have had more foolishness than anything else." Many expressed the view that "all of the midwives have started with much less experience than we really should have."

In both states, those who started practicing before a formal course and apprenticeship system developed say they would have welcomed the opportunity for structured training. Even though half the licensed lay midwives in Arizona were self-taught or had learned their vocation in the process of nurse training or apprenticeships, only one (whose license has been suspended for violating several of the regulations) favors deregulation. Similarly, nearly three-quarters of the unregulated lay midwives in the northeastern state would like to have a mandatory licensure program that would standardize training. Most of the rest favor a voluntary system.

The desire for more rigorous training has increased the midwives' interest in becoming certified nurse-midwives. Six of the 27 Arizona midwives have become certified nurse-midwives since the interviews were completed. Sixteen of the 23 northeastern midwives have considered doing so and 2 plan to do so. Training in nurse-midwifery is difficult to obtain, however, owing to high costs, burdensome family responsibilities, and lack of access; there is only one school in Arizona and none in the northeastern state, and most schools require individuals to be registered nurses before applying.

Most of the remaining midwives in both states do not want to become certified nurse-midwives. They argue that "midwifery is a profession in and of itself separate from nursing" and feel that much of nurse training at best is irrelevant and at worst would be "corrosive" to their independence and nonmedicalized philosophy. They recognize that few nurse-midwives have the freedom (either legally or practically) to conduct home births and fear that nurse training would socialize them to be subordinate to physicians rather than to act as independent practitioners. As an alternative, the midwives favor the development of direct entry midwifery schools that require no nursing training, such as are available in England.

THE UNDERLYING PHILOSOPHY

The congruence of beliefs about pregnancy and childbirth among lay midwives in both states is as striking as the divergence in their backgrounds. To some degree this might be explained by their similar choices of reading material. Almost all mentioned reading several of the popular "alternative" birth publications: Gaskin's *Spiritual Midwifery*, Davis's *Guide to Midwifery*, and the magazines *The Practicing Midwife*, *Mothering*, and *Special Delivery*. However, almost all midwives also mentioned relying on *Williams' Obstetrics* and medical journals which exposed them to the mainstream medical perspective on pregnancy and childbirth, even though they did not share it.

The widespread familiarity with medical literature, even in the nonregulating state where midwives have not had to pass a qualifying examination, belies the commonly held view of lay midwifery as a totally demedicalized childbirth alternative. Such a dichotomous perspective misses the more complex dimensions of the philosophy of modern lay midwives, summarized in figure 3.1. Rather than advocating a return to the questionable quality of care before the advent of obstetrics, the midwives believe that they are the harbingers of twenty-first-century obstetrics. They recognize the value of obstetrical science for managing the complications inevitably experienced by a small minority of pregnant women. All assert that they "couldn't practice without medical, professional, and hospital backup." At the

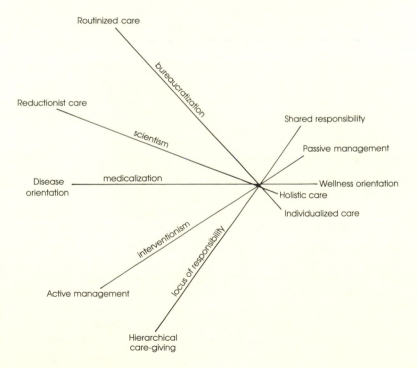

Figure 3.1 A Model of Midwifery Care

same time, they fear the physical and emotional dangers that arise when interventionist practices, developed for the pathological, become the obstetrical norm. In contrast, they strongly believe in the general normalcy of pregnancy and childbirth and in the benefits of individualized, holistic, and participatory maternity care.

WELLNESS ORIENTATION

When asked how their perspective on maternity care differs from that of obstetricians, the midwives compare the disease orientation of physicians to their own wellness orientation. As one says:

> Midwives have a really strong belief and faith in the natural process and the wisdom of that. Obviously it is not a blind faith because we are aware of the problems that develop. But on the whole, obstetricians tend to see pregnancy as an illness . . . and labor as being a very dangerous time.

Even the most sympathetic obstetricians, they feel, tend to "medicalize" pregnancy. One midwife who assisted a group of family practitioners at home births and published a home birth guidebook with them reports:

> There were still attitudinal and philosophical differences between us, as good a team as we were. . . . The midwife sees the passage of the baby through the birth canal as a healthy, positive experience that is good for both the mother and the baby. . . . The physician sees . . . a dangerous passage . . . full of pitfalls.

Most attribute the physicians' more pathological definition of pregnancy and childbirth to the general disease orientation of medical training and the physicians' exposure to higher risk clientele. One suggests that "all you need to do is look at an obstetrics textbook and you see how little [text] is spent on normal birth." Another notes that, whereas midwives work with a healthy population, physicians "don't screen out the women who smoke and weigh 300 pounds." Some think that physicians, owing to their socialization as healers, are bored by normal births and consequently search for potential problems which would justify active intervention. These interventions

may in turn produce other complications requiring further intervention and reinforcing physicians' belief in the danger of childbirth.

PASSIVE MANAGEMENT

The midwives object to physicians' routine use of interventionist
practices initially developed for emergencies in the active management of normal pregnancy and childbirth. They express concern
about the readiness of physicians to use clinical procedures such as
induction, rupture of amniotic membranes, and episiotomy to speed
up the natural process:

> [Obstetricians are] not as willing [as midwives] to let the natural process
> take its course. I've seen it. I've seen, "Well you're 42 weeks by date; see you
> in the hospital in the morning to induce your labor." It's like they're just too
> ready to get in there and do things. They're too ready to break the water.
> They're too ready to just do all their little things that they can do.

Another questions the routine use of analgesics as a substitute for
staff attention in hospitals:

> If you do anesthesia or hospital drugs of any kind, you're setting up a
> whole snowball mechanism which could end up a cesarean or forceps, just
> misery. Once you have that baby, the pain goes away and you've got the
> baby. . . . If you support women enough, they can do it, with very few
> exceptions.

Similarly, one of the foreign-trained midwives who previously
worked on a maternity ward objects to the routine use of drugs to
augment labors:

> We don't accelerate nothing. The doctors do. That is why they sometimes
> make mistakes. They start to give too much medication. They start the
> labor too fast and the heartbeat starts to jump, and starts to fail, and they
> start to make forceps.

In contrast, the midwives often claim that one of the "biggest lessons
I've had to learn is to sit on my hands and not do anything."

The midwives offer the rising U.S. cesarean rate, now one in five
(Taffel et al., 1985), and the slightly higher forceps rate as examples
of abuse of interventionist procedures. The U.S. rates, they note, are
more than double those of other developed countries, many of which

have lower infant mortality. Several midwives point out that women who deliver in teaching hospitals or who have private hospital insurance have even higher cesarean and forceps rates. One wonders, "If all you know is women who have had cesareans, I'm not sure what your chances are [for vaginal delivery]. . . . That scares me more than anything else." This same midwife adds that although hospitals have opened birthing rooms in response to consumer demands for less intervention, "the cesarean rate is still the same. . . . You want to know how cynical I am? Vbacs [vaginal births after cesareans] could increase the primary cesarean section rate because . . . then, what is the [reason not to cut]?"

While the midwives support passive management for normal births, they recognize the need for interventionist techniques when specific problems arise. They see themselves as "risk-screeners." For this reason, many will not accept clients who seek total nonintervention.

All the midwives make plans for transferring a client to a hospital if serious complications requiring medical attention develop. Those unrestricted by licensure laws deal with less serious complications themselves. If needed, they perform an episiotomy, suture a minor perineal tear, and administer an antihemorrhagic drug or intravenous fluids. The licensed midwives in Arizona have been prohibited from such interventions, but almost all believe that these skills should be part of a midwife's resources.

SHARED RESPONSIBILITY

Closely related to the issue of medicalization and intervention is the distribution of authority and responsibility between the pregnant woman and her caregiver. The traditional medical system demands that patients adopt the sick role (Parsons, 1951), relinquishing responsibility for their health and placing themselves under physicians' supervision and guidance. The midwives strongly object to this hierarchical distribution of responsibility:

> The obstetrician is more apt to manage the pregnancy, manage the labor, and deliver the baby. Most lay midwives that I know are much more of the attitude that they are a facilitator of the woman's process. They are there to

help and support her and to facilitate things, make suggestions as appropriate, but pretty much step back and let her do her thing; let her develop
her own style of giving birth.

In keeping with their wellness philosophy the midwives criticize
women who adopt the sick role just because they are pregnant. They
also criticize physicians who "are too ready to take the power that a
woman naturally gives to her care provider . . . [and who] manipu-
late to get that power." Another midwife stated:

> There is a certain power imbalance between physicians and clients which
> tends to create for people the feeling that they can't take responsibility for
> their health care on a daily level [such as] nutrition . . . [They feel] that they
> are in the hands of the physicians and that they really don't need to worry
> about much. So the empowerment is a really big [issue] for me. Every time
> I catch someone asking me to take care of them in subtle ways . . , I feel that
> I should return the power to them.

In some ways the midwives' views about prenatal care resemble
those of physicians. Like physicians, midwives emphasize the importance of diet, exercise, rest, and abstention from tobacco and alcohol.
Unlike physicians, however, they believe that the probability of
choosing a healthy lifestyle will be greatly increased if clients retain or
develop a sense of self-responsibility. The most common nonmedical
reason why midwives decline or terminate the care of a client is the
belief that the client is irresponsible. The midwives often refer to
themselves as teachers when asked to distinguish their prenatal care
from that of physicians. Many have a collection of books that they
lend to clients. Some also have their clients monitor and record their
own urine and weight to teach them about their health and that of
their babies. They urge them to be informed consumers. One describes how she asks her clients: "Well, what did the doctor say? What
did that mean? Why didn't you ask him? . . . Don't take my word for
it, look it up yourself. . . . This is not beyond you. You can learn what
it takes to have a baby and rear a baby. You don't have to go to
someone else."

The midwives want their clients involved in the birthing process as
well. They believe that if "the parents can reclaim control over the
birth experience that will make for a better outcome of the birth."
Almost all encourage the father to catch the baby, cut the umbilical

cord and generally participate in the birth. Some mention teaching the father how to palpate the baby, having the woman reach down and touch the baby's head after it crowns, or having the mother bring the baby up onto her stomach after the shoulders are born.

The midwives generally accept clients' preferences about birthing procedures and whom they want at the birth. Most, however, draw the line at requests that they fear might jeopardize the mother or baby. For example, one with a client interested in underwater birthing says, "I would be relieved if she forgot about that idea. . . . I always try to keep a humble attitude about new things. . . . But, I wouldn't. I would have to read a lot of good medical studies before I felt comfortable with [it]." Another midwife's client had an acupuncturist at her birth for pain relief who wanted to treat a subsequent postpartum hemorrhage with needles. The midwife says she was "not liberal enough for that" and said, "You can do whatever you want but I'm going to give her pitocin."

The midwives' language reflects their philosophy about parental responsibility. They are careful to refer to the women they attend as "clients" or "ladies" rather than "patients." One who used the term "patient" during an interview quickly corrected herself. Most describe their role as "catching" the baby "delivered" by the mother.

As the preceding examples illustrate, all midwives recognize that despite their commitment to nonhierarchical care, their role involves a great deal of responsibility. Although almost all say that the woman, the couple, or the couple together with the midwife have the basic responsibility for decisions about birthing procedures, the majority qualify this response with statements such as "when push comes to shove, it ends up being the midwife. You have to be prepared to take the responsibility."

In practice this means that midwives' clients have a great deal of control over how they labor—in a bathtub, on a bed, walking around, on their hands and knees, or however they feel comfortable. As long as things proceed normally, they also have a great deal of control over how they deliver—their support people, their position, whether they want Leboyer techniques, and so on. Reclaiming control over the birth experience is the central tenet of the home birth movement. But when a complication arises, such as a depressed baby, the midwives know that "there is no way [the parents] can digest enough material to make an informed choice." The midwives' role then changes from "watch dogs of the norm" to being trained emergency technicians.

HOLISTIC CARE

Besides defining childbirth as a potentially pathological process requiring active management, the medical perspective assumes that problems stem from specific organic factors. This reductionist view leads to an emphasis on the physical condition of a patient and downplays psychological and social factors. The midwives, in contrast, possess a holistic view that stresses the importance of psychological and social influences. As one puts it:

> I think we give a lot more attention to women as women and not just a growing uterus. . . . We talk to them in real detail, emotionally—how they are feeling with the pregnancy; how they are adjusting to all the changes; how they are doing in their relationship with their family; and how the pregnancy fits in with their life. We really try to work with them on many levels, physically, emotionally.

Experience has reinforced the midwives' belief in the importance of social and psychological factors. One, for example, told of a birth where she was convinced that the tension created by the unexpected arrival of the husband's previous wife during the delivery caused his current wife's retained placenta. The assisting physician could not dislodge the placenta and the woman had to be transferred to a hospital for manual removal.

The most commonly mentioned psychological factor affecting childbirth is confidence in one's ability to give birth without medical assistance. One generalized that "the uterus of a fearful woman just doesn't work very well." All the midwives occasionally get clients who have doubts about home birth. In some cases, their partners or friends have pressured them to have a home birth. In other cases, the woman is afraid of hospitals or wants to save money. The midwives have learned that such a woman is a poor risk for home birth and can "bleed like a sewer" because of the "power of the mind on the body."

Most midwives mention the importance of the relationship between the couple and between the couple and the midwife. Several also mention the importance of the woman's relationship with her mother and the need to discuss it prenatally. The midwives encourage their clients to bring their partners to prenatal visits. All make at least one prenatal home visit, which allows them to observe family dynamics as well as screen the planned birthing location.

To facilitate holistic care, the midwives schedule prenatal visits lasting from one-half to two hours. This, they point out, is in marked contrast with the typical "five minute" physician visit. While the midwives claim greater thoroughness in their physical assessment, they also readily admit that they spend most of the time teaching and counseling. Some have clients keep diaries that include personal feelings as well as notes on diet and physical complaints. Others have prenatal visit forms that ask about recent moods and fears so that they can be discussed. Some also use visualization techniques to create a positive attitude to labor and delivery.

INDIVIDUALIZED CARE

The midwives' attention to social and psychological as well as physical factors in pregnancy and birthing leads them to strive for a more individualized style of care. This goes beyond including clients in the decision-making process and being open to preferences about labor and delivery procedures. It extends to a belief that "you don't have one approach for all women and they have to fit your approach; you fit your approach to the woman."

The social and psychological information gathered during prenatal care is regarded as an "invaluable tool to have going into labor." The midwives draw on their familiarity with a particular client's strengths and weaknesses, fears, and desires to anticipate and stem potential problems and to facilitate preferences. They act as an emotional support person if the client's partner or chosen friend does not successfully fill that role.

The midwives' emphasis on individualized care does not mean a total absence of bureaucracy in their practices. Virtually all have adopted some routine record-keeping procedures. The licensed midwives must submit a standardized record of prenatal, labor, and delivery information for each client to the state regulatory department. All keep additional records of prenatal appointments and other information that they deem useful. Many record labor and delivery notes on forms similar to those used in hospitals. Although the nonregulated midwives are not legally bound to keep records, many keep records as detailed as those of the regulated midwives. In general, the larger a midwife's practice the more routinized is her record keeping.

The midwives recognize that a large clientele makes increased bureaucracy inevitable. Hence, all but a few limit their practice to two or three scheduled births per month. One of the exceptions, a licensed midwife, on occasion has had to rent motel rooms and call in other midwives so that she can attend several deliveries simultaneously. Although she takes pride in her successful business of more than 100 births per year, the other midwives have stigmatized her for no longer providing individualized, family-centered, holistic care. None has emulated her.

Even those who attend two to five births per month usually must reserve specific days for prenatal visits at the midwife's house and for prenatal screening and postpartum visits at clients' houses. Six of the licensed and two of the nonregulated midwives with practices of this size have set up offices in their homes or elsewhere with waiting and examining areas, including the three Mormon midwives who use their fully equipped clinic. Seven other licensed midwives provide prenatal care at a local "free clinic." The rest of the midwives make do with the unmodified informal setting of their own or clients' homes. In the past, however, approximately nine of these provided their prenatal care with a physician at the physician's office.

In addition to bureaucratizing records and care, some midwives have moved toward routinizing their collection of fees. Those who began practicing in the early to mid-1970s did not initially charge for their services. Over time, their compensation has evolved along with the size of their practices from the personal gratification of providing a valued service, through a stage of informal gifts and semiformal bartering, to a cash business. Most midwives admit that they have few skills in business, more quilts than they can use, and many bad debts. Although none is ready to assign her nonpaying clients to bill collection agencies as physicians do, attitudes about payment have changed over time. Initially many felt guilty about charging for a service to which they feel religiously or philosophically committed. Recognition that the personal time involved is time away from their own families and, in some cases, other jobs has offset this guilt. Moreover, the midwives need reinbursement for the many expenses incurred— babysitters, beepers, telephone answering service, transportation, equipment, and training workshop tuition. Some have come to view payment as an affirmation of the skills and quality of care provided as well. As a result, the longer a midwife practices, the likelier she is to phase out bartering for unneeded goods or services and to require at least half of her fee paid before the birth.

THE WOMEN'S PERSPECTIVE

In sum, the midwives believe that they differ from physicians in emphasizing the normality of childbirth, encouraging women to take responsibility for their own bodies, and providing holistic, individualized care with minimal intervention. The midwives feel that these differences in part reflect the fact that they are women whereas most physicians are men. Those midwives who have given birth state that their philosophy derives from their own experiences—experiences most obstetricians cannot share. The other midwives acquired their philosophy from close personal associations with women who had given birth. The midwives feel that these experiences confirmed their intuitive belief in the inherent normalcy of pregnancy and birth while making them more sensitive to, and sympathetic with, the "aches and pains" and "emotional changes that women experience during pregnancy and postpartum." They also feel that firsthand experience with birth has given them patience and respect for the couples' desires. The emphasis on personal experience as a qualification for midwifery has been so strong that midwives who are childless sometimes have felt unwelcome.

At the same time, some midwives believe that obstetricians' perspective on childbirth and style of care-giving reflect male sexism. They suspect that physicians lack respect for, and trust in, women's bodies and women's ability to understand their bodies. Midwives, they assert, "have a lot more respect for the women . . . [whereas] he thinks he knows more than her." (The midwives who bring up the issue of sexism note that female obstetricians do not usually differ greatly from their male counterparts, because of their socialization in the "male" world of medicine.)

The values underlying the midwives' perspective are values feminists have identified as typically female. Their style of practice is
more passive than active. The midwives trust nature with all its vari-
ability and intuition as well as science and logic. They believe that an
individual woman's feelings and personal experience more accurately reflect her progress in labor and delivery than do statistically
derived norms for how childbirth "should" proceed. And they believe in recognizing the value of, and dealing with, emotions and
interpersonal relationships rather than treating them as extraneous
factors or hindrances. This congruence between midwives' beliefs
and typically female values supports the midwives' view that their
philosophy and style of practice derive from their womanhood.

Yet none of the Arizona midwives and only six in the Northeast
became midwives as a consciously feminist response to male-domi-
nated obstetrics. In fact, the early feminist health movement was
sometimes unsympathetic to home birth. This view was reflected in
the first edition of *Our Bodies, Ourselves* (1971), as well as in the refusal
of a feminist health group to aid some of the northeastern midwives
in establishing a home birth service. These feminists wanted to break
the nuclear family's hold over women and recognized that the home
birth movement aimed to strengthen the family. Indeed, a strong
commitment to nurturing family bonds unites all midwives, feminists
and conservatives alike.

PRACTICE

The homogeneity of philosophy among lay midwives in the two states
has resulted in many similarities in their practices. Few midwives in
either state want to attend more than four scheduled births per
month because of their desire to provide individualized care. Nevertheless, the volume of clientele ranges from less than one to ten
births each month. The number of clients depends in part on how
long the midwife has been practicing, whether she has an additional
job, and, most important, the ages of her own children. Half the
midwives in the northeastern state and in Arizona had a child under
three at the time of the interview. Several had sharply curtailed their
practices or were phasing them out because of family responsibilities.

Some women who began attending home births in the mid-1970s

did not initially provide prenatal care because they did not then view themselves as midwives. All now require that their clients see them for prenatal care. The Arizona midwives by law must encourage their clients to seek additional prenatal care from a physician, and some of the unregulated midwives do this as well. Most see their clients an average of eight to ten times before the birth. They follow the usual obstetrical schedule of one visit per month until the last month or two and then every one or two weeks depending on nearness to the due date.

The prenatal examinations conducted by the regulated and unregulated midwives are strikingly similar. All keep charts on blood pressure, weight, blood and urine, fetal growth, and heartbeat—the standard obstetrical assessments. The rest of the one- or two-hour appointment is filled with discussions of nutrition and other holistic concerns.

All visit the client's house at least once to check conditions and supplies. Many stress the importance of this visit, which allows the family to become comfortable with the midwife's presence in their home. After the birth all make postpartum visits to monitor the health of mother and child.

Despite the overall similarities in practices between the two states, some notable differences exist as well. These stem from the different legal positions of midwives in Arizona and the northeastern state. The next two chapters discuss how contemporary American law deals with midwifery and how licensure has affected the practices of lay midwives.

REFERENCES

Boston Women's Health Book Collective. *Our Bodies, Ourselves*. Boston: Simon & Schuster, 1971.

Davis, Elizabeth. *A Guide to Midwifery: Heart and Hands*. Santa Fe: John Muir, 1981.

Gaskin, Ina May. *Spiritual Midwifery*. Summertown, TN: The Book Publishing Company, 1978.

Hellman, Louis, and Jack Pritchard. *Williams' Obstetrics*, 14th ed. London: Butterworth's, 1971.

Parsons, Talcott. *The Social System*. Glencoe, IL: Free Press, 1951.

Taffel, Selma, Paul Placek, and Mary Moien. "One Fifth of 1983 U.S. Births by Cesarean Section." *American Journal of Public Health* 75:190, 1985.

CHAPTER 4
THE LAW AND MIDWIFERY

It is difficult to ascertain the current legal status of lay midwives. Health care in the United States is still dominated by state regulation, and this fragmented control allows states considerable latitude in dealing with home birth midwives. Tracking midwives' legal status is particularly difficult since this is an area of active legislation and government officials sometimes disagree on the interpretation of relevant older laws and court cases. In addition, midwives' apparent legal position may bear little resemblance to their actual circumstances. Problems with enforcement may render legislation prohibiting midwifery impotent, and lenient midwifery licensing laws may be circumvented by state officials who indefinitely delay granting licenses.

According to a recent law review (Wolfson, 1986), lay midwifery was clearly legal in 11 states in 1986 (Alaska, Arizona, Mississippi, New Hampshire, New Jersey, New Mexico, South Carolina, Tennessee, Texas, Washington, and the six poorest counties in Arkansas). Lay midwifery is definitely illegal in ten states (Colorado, Connecticut, Delaware, Hawaii, Indiana, Maryland, Montana, New York, Pennsylvania, and West Virginia) and effectively illegal in another twelve states (Alabama, Georgia, Florida, Illinois, Kentucky, Louisiana, Minnesota, Missouri, North Carolina, Ohio, Rhode Island, and Virginia) that still have lenient, old "granny midwife" laws[1] on their books but no longer grant new licenses. In the remaining

---

1. These laws were passed in earlier years in many states to improve maternity care in poor and medically underserved areas.

states, no statute or court decision unequivocally addresses lay midwifery. In these circumstances, lay midwives' freedom to practice relies heavily on the politics and philosophies of prosecutors, judges, and regulatory boards (Throne and Hanson, 1981). Consequently, midwives' status in these states remains uncertain until either legislatures pass new laws or judges write new opinions on older laws defining the practice of medicine or certified nurse-midwifery.

States where lay midwifery is legal can be classified into three groups. Some, such as Alaska, Arizona, New Mexico, and South Carolina, have developed relatively rigorous licensure standards for those seeking to practice midwifery. Alternatively, states can merely register, rather than license, midwives or set only minimal requirements for practice. Texas, for example, until 1984 only required midwives to record their names, addresses, and occupation at their local courthouses. The state estimated that more than 400 lay midwives were practicing there when new regulations went into effect (personal communication, Texas Dept. of Health, 5/11/84). These new regulations state that midwives can attend only normal childbirth and cannot prescribe drugs or use surgical implements; they do not tighten the requirements for registration (Tex. Rev. Civ. Stat., 1983). Finally, two states, Mississippi and Tennessee, officially permit any individual to initiate a home birth practice and neither register nor license them.

Lay midwives unquestionably risk legal sanctions in states where laws or court decisions have been interpreted as defining attendance at births as the practice of medicine. The first court case of this sort against a midwife occurred in Massachusetts in 1907 (Commonwealth v. Porn) and is still cited in judicial opinions (Katz, 1980). Midwives have been arrested in recent years for practicing medicine without a license in California, Illinois, Missouri, Vermont, Colorado, Arkansas, and elsewhere (California Association of Midwives, 1983; Darrash, 1985; Lupa, 1985; Tjaden, 1982). Midwives in states without clear statutes or legal precedents also risk these legal charges, since prosecutors can at any time attempt to apply statutes regarding medical practice to midwifery.

Midwives also may face prosecution for child abuse, manslaughter, or homicide if a mother or infant suffers injury or death. Such cases have occurred in California, Texas, Illinois, and Michigan. George

Annas, a public health legal analyst, explains that "home birth offers the family and the birth attendant greater autonomy at the sacrifice of the legal umbrella of a hospital. Personnel and procedures not legitimized by the authority of a hospital will be subjected to stricter legal scrutiny in the event of a bad outcome" (1984:52). As a result, according to one commentator, "the unspoken legal rule of thumb appears to be: if a baby dies at home, the attending midwife will be charged with murder or a felony. If the baby dies in the hospital, it's an act of God" (Fitzgerald, 1980:33).

The threat of indictment serves as a powerful disincentive to midwifery. One woman we interviewed, for example, in a state where midwifery was of questionable legality, said:

> My daughter's worried about me going to jail. I don't like her having to worry about that. . . . I got stopped for speeding on my way to a birth and [my daughter] was in the back seat with my bags. She threw a blanket over the bags and sat on them. . . . It bothers the hell out of me. I get very paranoid when I have to take a woman to the hospital. I am scared to death I'm going to get busted. I don't want to go to jail.

Although working within regulatory guidelines gives licensed and registered midwives some protection against legal charges, their marginal social status may still leave them vulnerable to prosecution. As one licensed midwife described:

> Unlicensed midwives in other states are worried all the time for getting in trouble for practicing because they're not licensed. Licensed midwives have . . . the same problems because we have to submit reports and so forth and because it seems the Department of Health Services hears about every little thing. We worry all the time that they're gonna come along and bust us for some little minor infringement. We're all aware that the Department of Health Services has a big fat file on every single one of us and that every small transgression's on that file. . . . And the little, little things they never say anything about until you do something that is half way major and then they're gonna pull out the whole list. . . . It's just a whole different paranoia [from being unlicensed], but the paranoia's still there.

MIDWIFERY IN THE COURTS

As midwifery's popularity has grown in every state, regardless of legal status, so have the number of court cases brought against lay midwives. In California, where midwifery is widespread, at least 19 lay midwives were charged with practicing medicine without a license between 1974 and late 1983, and 4 of these were additionally indicted for murder or manslaughter (California Association of Midwives, 1983).

Home birth proponents assert that most prosecutions of lay midwives stem from physicians' desire to protect their authority and monopoly rather than from consumer complaints about quality of care or public concern about safety or law-breaking (DeVries, 1985:121–29). For example, midwife Marianne Doshi's 1978 arrest in California for murder and practicing medicine without a license was instigated by the chief of obstetrics at a local hospital. Doshi had transported to the hospital a newborn who had been born with a true knot in the umbilical cord and serious breathing problems. The judge dismissed the charges following a pretrial hearing in which the parents praised the midwife's resuscitation of the infant. He commented for the record, "I am convinced . . . that had that child died in the hospital, or at home under a doctor's care, that we would have a thousand doctors lined up between here and Los Angeles willing to testify that the doctor provided medical treatment according to the standard of care" (quoted in DeVries, 1985:123).

Another well-publicized legal case in California demonstrates the various legal hazards midwives face. Rosalie Tarpening was arrested after the 1979 birth of a baby who died, according to the coroner's report, from aspiration of amniotic fluid and subarachnoid hemorrhage (Bowers, 1981b). Tarpening, a licensed physical therapist and lay midwife, claimed to have been the primary attendant at 354 deliveries over a nine-year period with no previous fetal or newborn deaths and no need to transport mothers or infants to a hospital (Bowers, 1981a). She was charged initially with first-degree murder (which carries a mandatory death sentence in California), practicing medicine without a license, and grand theft for charging for her services. She spent seven days in jail before her bail was lowered from $100,000 to $25,000 and she could mortgage her home to raise the bond. During the preliminary hearings over the next two years, the prosecution contended that Tarpening had caused the death through mismanagement of labor resulting in insufficient oxygen. The defense argued that the baby died because the physicians at the receiving hospital pushed air into the baby's lungs at too great a pressure in their resuscitation attempt. Although the case was controversial among midwives, the California Association of Midwives formally proclaimed their support for Tarpening, as did the founder of Informed Homebirth (Baldwin, 1980). A judge dismissed the murder charge for lack of the required evidence of malicious intent each of the three times it was filed by the prosecutor.

Tarpening eventually was tried only for practicing medicine without a license. In spite of the defense's attempts, the judge refused to permit expert witnesses to testify regarding the safety of home births. The jury found Tarpening guilty. She received a one-year suspended jail sentence, on the stipulation that she attend no births in any capacity during the next two years. Although her sentence was minimal, Tarpening had lost thousands of dollars and two years of her life in fighting these charges. In addition, the state licensing board suspended her physical therapist license for six months, depriving her of her main source of income.

As these examples demonstrate, lay midwives occupy a legally vulnerable position. Practical difficulties blunt the potential force of the law, however. Home birth parents have made a voluntary choice of a radical alternative. Even in those rare instances when infants die, the parents almost always believe that the midwife provided care superior to that obtainable from an obstetrician and, consequently, refuse to swear out a complaint. When physicians initiate complaints, the parents usually defend the midwife's actions.

Lack of consumer cooperation has led a few police agencies to adopt tactics similar to those used in other victimless crimes when pressured by prosecutors to stop midwifery activity. The California State Department of Consumer Affairs, for example, sent a pregnant undercover agent to solicit the services of several Santa Cruz midwives in 1974 (Arms, 1975), and undercover police officers in Illinois approached a midwife about having a home birth in 1983 (NAPSAC News, 1983a:7). These midwives subsequently were charged with practicing medicine without a license. Although such actions are a constant fear among midwives practicing without the protection of licensure, they have been rare, probably because they raise the controversial legal issue of entrapment.

Since parents generally support their midwives, prosecutors have had little success arguing that midwives' actions constitute malicious intent or negligence. As a result, most cases that come to trial involve only the philosophically controversial issue of whether midwifery is the practice of medicine. Physician authority on this issue is weakened by their obvious conflict of interest and judicial outcomes have been mixed. In the 19 California cases, 9 midwives either had all charges dropped or won acquittals; the other 10 were convicted of practicing medicine without a license. To date, no midwife has been convicted of murder or manslaughter anywhere in the country. As DeVries (1985:136–37) notes, the fact that few unlicensed midwives have been sentenced to jail suggests that the courts regard the available punishments as overly severe.

Criminal prosecution is not the only legal risk midwives face, however. Midwives, such as Rosalie Tarpening, who are licensed in another health care field expose themselves to disciplinary action by these boards in addition to, or even in the absence of, legal prosecution. In 1982, Janet Leigh, a registered nurse and lay midwife, came to the attention of her nursing board following a planned home birth in which the fetus' umbilical cord prolapsed, becoming caught in the vagina and cutting off its oxygen supply (Knox, 1983). The midwife called an ambulance to take the woman to the hospital for an emergency cesarean section. Although the ambulance personnel were untrained in childbirth, they refused to allow the midwife to continue the standard intervention needed to maintain the fetus's blood and oxygen supply, despite her frantic protests. The infant died following a hospital delivery. This same hospital twice previously had suspended Leigh's nursing privileges because of her home birth activities. After the infant death, the chief obstetrical nurse brought a complaint to the State Board of Registration in Nursing against Leigh, alleging that she had dishonestly described herself as a certified nurse-midwife to the emergency medical technicians.

The board suspended Leigh's license for misrepresenting herself as a certified nurse-midwife and for "gross misconduct in the practice of nursing" (Knox, 1984). No specific misconduct was mentioned, but the decision cited the 1907 case defining midwifery as the practice of medicine and noted that Massachusetts law prohibits certified nurse-midwives from attending home births.

Leigh appealed this decision in state court. Testimony by physicians at the trial indicated that she had given appropriate care until prevented by the emergency medical technicians. No one argued that Leigh's actions contributed to the infant's death. Under cross-examination, the technicians admitted that during their argument with her, Leigh may have referred to herself initially as a nurse and later as a midwife rather than as a certified nurse-midwife. The judge ordered the board to justify its decision better. The board then deleted the charge that Leigh misrepresented her training but specified that conducting home births and working as a midwife without certification in nurse-midwifery constituted gross misconduct for a registered nurse. In a subsequent rehearing, the State Supreme Court concluded that midwifery does not constitute the practice of medicine but that the Board of Registration in Nursing has the right to discipline nurses who disobey its guidelines (Leigh v. Board of Registration in Nursing, 1985). As a result of this decision, any lay midwife, except those who are also registered nurses, now may practice legally in Massachusetts.

The irony of this situation did not go unnoticed. In response, a bill was proposed in the 1986 legislative session that would establish a Board of Midwifery to regulate and license lay midwives and allow registered nurses to become licensed as lay midwives without jeopardizing their nursing credentials. Previous legislative attempts to establish lay midwifery licensure in Massachusetts had failed due to widespread physician opposition and legislators' hesitancy to support alternative health care practitioners in a state that prides itself on having the highest per capita distribution of physicians (U.S. Bureau of the Census, 1984:103). The current bill's chances of passing, however, are better than previous bills. Many legislators now feel that, if midwifery is legal, it should be regulated and that it is illogical to open midwifery to all but registered nurses.

Legal treatment of registered nurses who practice midwifery provides a good example of the vast differences among state laws. A case in Tennessee similar to that of Janet Leigh's resulted in the opposite conclusion. The court found that if midwifery is legal, it cannot be considered misconduct in nursing (Leggett v. Tennessee Board of Nursing, 1981).

Another potential legal hazard of lay midwifery practice is the possibility of receiving civil injunctions or restraining orders from state regulatory agencies (Tjaden, 1982). Such actions have taken place in Arizona, Massachusetts, Colorado, and probably elsewhere. Midwives who ignore these orders may face fines or jail terms on contempt charges.

A final legal risk to lay midwives comes from the possibility of civil suits for malpractice. Our search of legal and other sources through 1986 found only three such cases. The paucity of such suits testifies to the loyalty of midwives' clients and their commitment to home birth. This stands in sharp contrast to the experience of obstetricians, 60 percent of whom have been sued for malpractice (Casselberry, 1985:630).

A current case from El Paso, Texas, is the most significant of the three exceptions. Until very recently, unregulated lay midwifery was an accepted part of Texas life. The visibility of lay midwifery in the city of El Paso was exceptionally high due to the presence of the midwife-run, nonprofit Alameda Maternity Center. The midwives at this center conducted 8,500 births in the last decade, primarily among poor Mexican immigrants. The city government's concern about their practice grew after a maternal death from postpartum hemorrhage in 1980 (Zamarripa, March 18, 1985). As a result, El Paso instituted its own regulations and established a Lay Midwifery Commission to enforce them. They now require lay midwives to pass an examination before practicing, restrict their practice to low risk groups, and consult a physician if certain specified complications arise (Palmer, 1985).

Despite these additional safeguards, a second woman, Sofia Rangel, bled to death in February 1985 following the birth of a healthy infant at the center. Rangel had gone to the center for care because the local county hospital does not provide prenatal care to illegal aliens (Zamarripa, March 7, 1985). After the death, Velia Rodriguez, Rangel's midwife and the director of the center, was arrested and charged with involuntary manslaughter. A subcommittee of the Lay Midwifery Commission revoked her license temporarily and recommended permanent revocation. They contended that Rodriguez, who claims to have attended about 9,000 births in Texas and Mexico over the last 31 years without a death, violated regulations when she did not consult a physician despite Rangel's severe tear from vagina to rectum and profuse bleeding. Instead, also in

violation of the newly enacted regulations, the midwife had attempted to suture the tear before taking the woman to a hospital
(personal communication, El Paso Lay Midwifery Commission,
1986). According to newspaper accounts, Rangel's mother claimed
that the midwife and her two assistants pressed on her daughter's
abdomen to push the infant out and refused her pleas that they take
her daughter to a physician (Zamarripa, March 15, 1985). The attending midwives, on the other hand, claimed that Rangel's blood
loss was unexceptional, that no external force was used, and that no
request was made to move her to the hospital (personal communication, Alameda Maternity Center, May 1986). Instead, they argued
that an unpreventable amniotic embolism killed Rangel when amniotic fluid entered her bloodstream. The coroner's report blamed
the death on "hypovolemic shock due to massive external bleeding
from a 4th degree [vagina to anus] tear of the perineum due to
delivery. The tear was very extensive and clearly visible from the
outside." Although evidence indicated an amniotic embolism, the
report noted that "the delay in seeking expert medical attention decreased the chances of survival." Rangel's family has filed a civil
damage suit for $1.7 million against the midwife, her two assistants,
the center's Board of Directors, and Shari Daniels, the lay midwife
who helped start the center. Less than two months later, another
malpractice suit was filed against several of the same individuals following a stillbirth (Heild, 1985). Daniels has since left the country,
while Rodriguez was convicted of involuntary manslaughter in the
Rangel case and sentenced to 10 years probation and a $5,000 fine.
The civil suits are still pending at the time of this writing.

THE LEGAL CASE FOR AND AGAINST LAY MIDWIFERY

The midwives' case for legalization rests upon constitutionally im-
plied rights to privacy and freedom of choice and upon a definition
of normal childbirth as outside the field of medicine. In all states,
women legally may choose to give birth at home (Annas, 1984; Wolfson, 1986). This is an empty choice, however, if they cannot obtain
trained attendants. The Association for Childbirth at Home International concluded, based on a small telephone survey and 441 un-
solicited letters it had received, that 61 percent of those who chose an

unattended home birth did so because no attendants were available (Brooks, 1979). Nothing obligates physicians to provide care and very few choose to attend home births. Physicians who refuse to provide care for home births, even in emergency situations, have not been held negligent by the courts. In a 1961 Louisiana case (Vindrine v. Mayes), an infant died after a home birth when all three physicians who were called refused to provide emergency care.

Although perhaps more certified nurse-midwives than physicians would like to conduct home births, they cannot do so legally without the approval of a supervising physician, and cannot do so at all in Massachusetts and Alabama. In a 1982 survey, 14 percent of certified nurse-midwives in the United States reported attending one or more home births (American College of Nurse-Midwives, 1984); this number decreased drastically in 1985 when nurse-midwives lost access to malpractice insurance for out-of-hospital work (as chap. 7 will discuss).

A significant test of whether the right to privacy applies to lay midwifery came in a 1976 California Supreme Court case (Bowland v. Municipal Court). The defendant midwives argued that laws against lay midwifery which de facto restrict choice of birth attendant and setting violate pregnant women's constitutional right to privacy. The court found against the midwives on the grounds that the state has a compelling interest in protecting the health of unborn children. Legal analysts criticized this decision sharply, contending that it insufficiently acknowledged recent extensions of privacy rights to families (Caldwell, 1983; Tachera, 1980). Additionally, they argued that the court had assumed without evidence that home birth is unnecessarily dangerous and that women choose home birth without regard for their children's best interests, since the court had based its decision on abortion law, where the interest of mother and embryo are obviously antithetical.

A class action suit in Illinois attempted to force the state to reestablish midwifery licensing on the grounds of privacy rights and discrimination. Illinois had granted midwife licenses until 1965, when a new statute ended that program. In 1977, ten pregnant women wishing a midwife-attended home birth and eleven women desiring licensing filed suit against the state. The mothers claimed violation of their constitutional privacy rights, while the midwives argued they were being denied equal protection since the law favored certified nurse-midwives and physicians over lay midwives. The judge dismissed the suit on the grounds that he "couldn't sec-ond-guess the motivation of the Illinois legislature in discontinuing midwifery licensure" (Davis, 1979:611).

At the crux of the legal argument for lay midwifery is the belief that childbirth is a natural process rather than a disease. By extension, attending normal labors and deliveries cannot constitute the practice of medicine. In most circumstances, the difference between a disease and a natural, normal physiological function seems obvious. In a highly medicalized society like the United States, however, this dis-tinction is less clear (Tjaden, 1982). Laws which do not define the difference merely reflect the monopolistic authority that American society since the first half of the twentieth century has given to physi-cians to define the scope of their autonomous profession. The mid-wives' legal case is damaged further by the fact that, while they seek to provide "well-women" care, they also must search for and diagnose any abnormalities that would preclude their continued involvement as primary caregivers. Even more ambiguous are the activities of some midwives who cut emergency episiotomies, suture tears, and administer antihemorrhagic drugs, all of which are usually regarded as medical treatments.

Federal law provides no help in this definitional debate; each state defines the practice of medicine as it chooses (Katz, 1980). The devel-opment of such definitions readily becomes the occasion for political battles between groups with conflicting interests. State laws differ so dramatically because the bargaining power of medical, nursing, mid-wifery, and consumer groups varies widely across the country. Na-tionally, however, medical associations are powerful lobbies; during the 1981–82 election cycle, for example, the American Medical Asso-ciation and its California and Texas branches comprised three of the top four contributors to political campaigns among business and pro-fessional Political Action Committees (NAPSAC News, 1983b:24).

DEVELOPMENT OF MIDWIFERY LAWS IN ARIZONA

The situation in Arizona demonstrates the political struggles under-lying midwifery regulation (Weitz and Sullivan, 1986). Arizona, like several other states such as New Mexico, Washington, and Texas, had never repealed its 1957 "granny midwife" law. Laws of this sort were passed in many states early this century. Because of Arizona's late development, it was one of the last states to pass such a law. To become a midwife, a woman needed only to know the fundamentals of hygiene, have basic (and unspecified) knowledge of the mechanics of labor and delivery, and be able to read and write English. This law gradually fell into disuse over the next twenty years. By the early 1970s, only three women, who practiced together in an isolated, polygamous Mormon town with no nearby physicians, still held active licenses.

During the 1970s, in Arizona as elsewhere, the burgeoning maternity rights movement led to the emergence of the new generation of lay midwives. In 1977, pressure from local physicians led the attorney general's office to prosecute one of these illegal midwives. The midwife's lawyer discovered the 1957 licensure law while researching her case. Because the midwife was a registered nurse, she easily met the requirements for licensing. To avoid a countersuit, the Department of Health Services decided to grant her a license and to consider other pending requests for licenses. This opened the door for nine other practicing midwives in the state to become licensed after passing a written, oral, and clinical qualifying examination and without any formal coursework.

Neither the Department of Health Services nor the state medical community approved of the resurgence of lay midwifery and the reactivation of the licensure program. Physicians responded by lobbying the legislature to make midwifery illegal, but Arizona has a long history of supporting free trade and opposing regulation and these efforts proved unsuccessful. Recognizing that legal lay midwifery would continue, the Department of Health Services adopted more stringent rules and regulations in 1978. Retention of these regulations has been difficult, since the department must constantly fight the legislature's antiregulatory philosophy. When unlicensed midwives' complained to sympathetic legislators that the absence of educational programs in Arizona made it impossible for them to qualify for licenses without leaving the state, the legislature approved a one-year grace period (1982/83) during which requirements were loosened. As this example demonstrates, Arizona midwives have retained a surprising degree of legal support for their right to practice, in contrast to many other states. How they can practice, however, is tightly regulated, as the next chapter will show.

THE LAW, MIDWIFERY, AND GENDER

Although the social position of midwives has varied greatly over time and space, female midwives everywhere have shared the handicap of gender. Eighteenth- and nineteenth-century midwives worked to improve their position in Western societies that held little respect for women's intellectual abilities or physical stamina. Consequently, midwifery developed along two paths, differentiated by gender. Male midwives assimilated into the developing, largely male, and more prestigious medical profession. Female midwives remained a separate occupation or were cast together with nurses and destined to work under physician supervision.

In the United States, as in other Western societies, female midwives' ability to lobby effectively on their own behalf was severely limited by their legal and economic disfranchisement as women. In most states until the late nineteenth century, married women fell under their husbands' guardianship and had no independent legal status. Not until 1920 did women win the right to vote and, consequently, have some say in government policy. Social norms have been still slower to change; sex discrimination in admissions to educational programs, hiring and firing, and wages were rarely questioned before the 1970s.

Although contemporary American midwives no longer work under such extreme legal restrictions, gender norms continue to hamper midwives' quest for professional recognition. Lay midwives are fighting for a level of functional autonomy granted to no other "female" occupation. Nurses, social workers, teachers, and clerical workers almost always labor under direct or indirect control of "male" occupations. The few men entering these traditionally female occupations tend to rise rapidly to supervisory positions. As yet, too few women have passed through the window of opportunity to traditionally male occupations, provided by the antidiscrimination policies of the 1970s, to judge the impact on these occupations' status. The remaining employed women work in pink collar occupations such as hairstyling, which society has never considered important enough to justify male concern.

The male gender of most physicians significantly increases their credibility and lobbying power in the legal and judicial systems, which continue to be dominated by men. At the same time, the female gender of most midwives works against them. Moreover, the fact that it is women who are encroaching on their occupational turf appears to threaten physicians' egos and heighten their hostility. Previous research has shown that physicians were far more antagonistic to the development of nurse-practitioners than to the development of similarly trained, but generally male, physician assistants (Fottler, 1979) because the former, but not the latter, challenge physicians' gender-based authority. Perhaps midwifery's best hope of acceptance is the continuing increase in women physicians, which may reduce the differences in status, lobbying power, and vested interests between these two fields.

REFERENCES

American College of Nurse-Midwives. *Nurse-Midwifery in the United States: 1982*. Washington, DC: 1984.

Annas, George. "Legal aspects of home birth," pp. 51–64 in Stanley E. Sagov, Richard F. Feinbloom, and Peggy Spindel (eds.), *Home Birth*. Rockville, MD: Aspen Systems, 1984.

Arms, Suzanne. *Immaculate Deception*. Boston: Houghton Mifflin, 1975.

Baldwin, Rahima. "A call for unity and support." *Special Delivery* 3:3, 1980.

Bowers, John B. "Tarpening case concluded." *NAPSAC News* 6:8–9, 1981[a].

Bowers, John B. "Homebirth on trial: The Rosalie Tarpening hearing." *Mothering*, pp. 69–77, Spring 1981[b].

Bowland v. Municipal Court, 134 Cal. Rptr. 630 (1976).

Brooks, Tonya. "Unattended home births," pp. 517–21 in David Stewart and Lee Stewart (eds.), *Compulsory Hospitalization*, Vol. 2. Marble Hill, MO: NAPSAC Reproductions, 1979.

Caldwell, Harry M. "Bowland v. Muncipal Court Revisited: A defense perspective on unlicensed midwife practice in California." *Pacific Law Journal* 15:19–33, 1983.

California Association of Midwives. "Midwives and other outlaws," unpublished paper. 1983.

Casselberry, Ellen. "Forum on malpractice issues in childbirth." *Public Health Reports* 100:629–33, 1985.

Commonwealth v. Porn, 82 N.E. 31 (Mass. 1907).

Darrash, Ida. "Midwifery in Arkansas." *MANA News* 3:1+, 1985.

Davis, Hope V. "The making of an educated lay midwife and my encounter with the law," pp. 603–12 in David Stewart and Lee Stewart (eds.), *Compulsory Hospitalization*, vol. 2. Marble Hill, MO: NAPSAC Reproductions, 1979.

DeVries, Raymond. *Regulating Birth: Midwives, Medicine and the Law.* Philadelphia: Temple University Press, 1985.

Fitzgerald, Linda. "Home birth: An alternative on trial." *New Age* 6:30–39, 1980.

Fottler, Myron D. "Physician attitudes toward physician extenders: A comparison of nurse practitioners and physician assistants." *Medical Care* 17:536–49, 1979.

Heild, Colleen. "Woman sues over baby's death." *El Paso Times,* p. 4-B, April 5, 1985.

Katz, Barbara F. "Childbirth and the law." *Colorado Medicine* 77:64–68, 1980.

Knox, Richard A. "Midwifery at issue in RN license case." *Boston Globe,* pp. 15+, October 14, 1983.

Knox, Richard A. "Midwife's RN license suspended." *Boston Globe,* pp. 21+, January 29, 1984.

Leggett v. Tennessee Board of Nursing, 612 S.W. 2d 476 (1981).

Leigh v. Board of Registration in Nursing, 481 N.E. 2d 1347 (Mass. 1985).

Lupa, Karen. "Midwest Region Report." *MANA News* 3:9, 1985.

NAPSAC News. "Midwifery in transition." 8:1–16, 1983a.

NAPSAC News. "Medical groups are largest political spenders." 8:24, 1983b.

Palmer, T. M. "Midwifery panel toughens ordinance to boost credibility." *El Paso Times,* p. 1+, June 12, 1985.

Tachera, Jennifer J. "A 'Birth Right': Home births, midwives and the right to privacy." *Pacific Law Journal* 12:97–119, 1980.

Tex. Rev. Civ. Stat. Ann. Art. 4512 (Vernon, 1983).

Throne, Linda J., and Lawrence P. Hanson. "Midwifery laws in the United States." *Women and Health* 6:7–26, 1981.

Tjaden, Patricia. "Homebirths, lay midwifery and the law." Paper presented at the American Society of Criminology meetings, Toronto, Ontario, 1982.

U. S. Bureau of the Census. *Statistical Abstract of the United States: 1985* (105th edition). Washington, DC: U.S. Government Printing Office, 1984.

Vindrine v. Mayes, 127 So. 2d 809 (Ct. Appl. La. 1961).

Weitz, Rose, and Deborah A. Sullivan. "The politics of childbirth: The re-emergence of midwifery in Arizona." *Social Problems* 33:163–75, 1986.

Wolfson, Charles. "Midwives and home birth: Social, medical and legal perspectives." *Hastings Law Journal* 37:909–67, 1986.

Zamarripa, Leticia. "How a midwife delivery turned into tragedy." *El Paso Herald-Post*, p. 1+, March 7, 1985[a].

Zamarripa, Leticia. "Police arrest midwife in 18-year-old's death." *El Paso Herald-Post*, pp. 1–2, March 15, 1985[b].

Zamarripa, Leticia. "Medical sector abuzz again over midwifery." *El Paso Herald-Post*, pp. 1–2, March 18, 1985[c].

CHAPTER 5
EFFECTS OF LICENSURE

Since the late 1970s state legislatures across the United States have debated the desirability of licensing lay midwives. For the most part, the chambers have echoed with the same questions heard at the turn of the century: Does the state's interest in the welfare of its citizens outweigh the right to privacy and free choice? To what extent is childbirth pathological and, consequently, a medical event? Can nonphysicians and non-nurses provide safe assistance at childbirth? This time, however, the lobby to license lay midwives has been led by the midwives and their ardent consumer supporters, not by physicians or public health officials.

The change in the proponents of midwifery licensure is significant. The external drive to license midwives in the early twentieth century resulted in restrictive and subordinating legislation that some social analysts (Anisef and Basson, 1979; Devitt, 1979; DeVries, 1985) feel helped to undermine the occupation. Such legislation has been described as a classic example of the corrosive effect of hostile licensure (DeVries, 1985:29). Nevertheless, midwives themselves are now seeking restrictive legislation with the hope of achieving legal recognition and protection and enhanced occupational status.

In advocating tighter control, the new midwifery licensure lobby is trying to follow the path to professional status that physicians blazed several decades ago. Midwives and their supporters recognize that the educational requirements, code of ethics, and standards of practice developed by physicians and institutionalized in licensing legislation have resulted in unparalleled social and economic status for this once-disparaged occupation. The midwives assume that by taking the lead in the legislative process they also can win a friendly licensure system that will improve their relationship with the medical system while removing the threat of prosecution for illegal activity. The only reservations that most unlicensed midwives have about licensure is the extent to which legal restrictions will hamper their practices.

EXPECTATIONS

Nearly three-quarters of the unlicensed midwives interviewed in the northeastern state favor a licensure program for lay midwives. They want licensure in order to practice openly—to advertise, to apply for third-party insurance payments, to obtain malpractice insurance, to have access to supplies, to consult with physicians, and to transfer problem cases to hospitals—without fear of prosecution. They believe that an open practice will allow them to reach women who are disenchanted with obstetrically managed normal births but unaware of any alternatives. They assume that the credibility of licensure will improve their rapport with physicians and hospital staff, enlarge the pool of physicians willing to provide backup, and smooth the way for hospital transfers when problems develop. One even foresees the possibility that licensure will open the door to hospital privileges for lay midwives. This midwife does not want to do planned hospital births but, like many others, would like to be able to "continue caring for my women" when hospital facilities prove needed. Without licensure she feels that she has no control and is "at the mercy of the obstetrician, . . . the pediatrician, [and] . . . the nursing staff."

Other anticipated benefits of licensure, mentioned by most of the more experienced unlicensed midwives, are regulation of midwifery training and the establishment of standards of care. Glossing over their own minimal initial qualifications, they complain that some newer midwives lack sufficient training to handle complications and caution in accepting potentially difficult cases. They feel that a few midwives are jeopardizing all midwives in the state by taking chances that engender medical opposition. As evidence, they point to high risk women who had been turned down for home birth by more experienced midwives but were subsequently attended by less experienced or out-of-state midwives. At least one such case, involving a woman who had previously had a cesarean, resulted in a perinatal death and unfavorable publicity for unlicensed midwives. Several other controversial perinatal deaths also have occurred in the last few years. One midwife tells of an unpromising apprentice whom she fired who

> went off on her own and started calling herself a midwife. She did a birth 20 miles from here and the baby died through her own incompetence. Ever since then, all the doctors around here think I was the midwife who did that. I would like to keep people like her out. . . . It reflects on all of us when somebody does something incompetent.

The reputation of unlicensed midwives also has been harmed by several less serious problem cases. Several midwives mention an incident, which occurred shortly before the interviews, in which two less experienced midwives called an ambulance when a client had a postpartum hemorrhage and then refused to allow the emergency medical personnel to enter the house. Instead, they requested that the paramedics stand by as a precaution while the midwives tried to manage the complication. Such controversial cases have forced the midwives to recognize that their reputations are tied to the practices of all others who call themselves midwives. Many agree with the midwife who asserts that most of the problems in her state "have been with midwives that I don't consider to be midwives but they consider themselves to be."

The less experienced midwives are more likely than the others to express mixed or negative views about licensure or other regulation. One acknowledges that "I'm quite sure, unfortunately, that there may be some midwives out there who are willing to do things that I would never do at home . . . [but] I don't want a mass organization where I have to answer to somebody."

To varying extents, most of the less experienced midwives cite philosophical objections to licensure and, more generally, professionalization. As one put it, licensure "takes away the responsibility from the consumer. . . . I feel that people should be able to get whatever kind of health care they want from anybody they want, and it's their responsibility to find out whether that person is capable." One highly experienced midwife, who also opposed licensure, cited George Bernard Shaw's idea (1930:107) that "all professions are a conspiracy against the laity" since they restrict the flow of knowledge.

She sees this territorial claim to knowledge and tools as antithetical to lay midwifery's emphasis on self-responsibility. This same midwife does not object to voluntary apprenticeship programs, examinations, or certification but argues that "licensing has always existed . . . to protect the interests of the practitioners, not the consumers." Another midwife argues more radically against any certification, titles, or degrees because

> "anyone can learn. . . . If you have knowledge . . . spread that knowledge . . . to as many people as you can. Not only will they benefit by it, but you'll benefit from them because they are coming at you in a whole different light. . . . [Restricting knowledge to those with degrees] is the same thing that doctors do to us.

At the time of the interviews, a few of the more experienced unlicensed midwives, with support from many others, were developing a voluntary certification program. Their aim is to "write our own rules before someone else writes them for us." They believe that regulation is inevitable and assume that a credible self-regulatory program would have a good chance of legislative adoption. To obtain a credential under their system, one must complete a prescribed training course and lengthy apprenticeship, demonstrate competence, be approved by three midwives with whom one has not trained, and agree to work within set screening criteria and other practice standards.

Unlicensed midwives in other states, such as Colorado, Idaho, and Texas, also are currently implementing credential programs. In addition, the Midwives Alliance of North America, a voluntary organization of certified nurse- and lay midwives, has proposed developing a North American Registry of Midwives (*MANA News*, 1987:2). To become registered, midwives generally will have to be licensed or certified in their state and then additionally pass a standardized examination which the association is currently developing.

All the midwives in the northeastern state support the concept of a voluntary credential program. Several of those who have mixed or negative feelings about licensure also have mixed feelings about the structure of this program, however. One of the critics suggests:

> It is very much a power struggle. . . . They want to charge $250 per birth to come and supervise me. . . . [The program] has been very effective in pushing out a number of people who can't afford that. They have done, in

effect, what the medical profession did to midwives a number of years ago. Here it is midwives doing it to other midwives.

The few with strong reservations about the voluntary certification program question not only the fees involved but also the assumption that the more experienced midwives, who began practicing with very little training, have the right to act as gatekeepers to midwifery. They further argue that some of the skills considered for inclusion, such as intubation and manual removal of the placenta, are too medical for a midwife's practice.

All of those with mixed or negative views on licensure, as well as many of those with positive views, worry about the effect that licensure might have on their practices. They fear that the loss of freedom will undermine their status as an alternative:

> People hope that it is going to be protection for them, whereas what actually happens in a lot of cases is that their hands are tied. . . . One of the reasons why people often choose to have a midwife is that they feel a midwife is more flexible and is able to provide them alternatives to the kind of protocols that their doctors often have. . . . Now, if midwives, by being certified, are ordered to follow the same protocols that doctors are following, then they are not offering the alternative that people are often in need of. If [the midwives] don't follow this protocol, whether they agree with it or not, then [the administrators] can cut off your nose to spite your face. You have a lot more to lose.

Some also worry about becoming "too professionalized":

> There is kind of a loyalty to the system or to the institution, or to their peers, or whatever. It somehow gets so out-of-hand that it overrides all your sympathy and your identification with the people you are serving. They aren't serving the people, they are serving the institution.

Another who is contemplating quitting midwifery expresses concern that as she and her partner becomes more knowledgeable and aware of the possible complications, they are losing their full commitment to shared responsibility in the delivery of maternity care and are adopting a more hierarchical style. She has observed several times when her partner "hasn't explained something [to their client] before she's done it. . . . Without giving them that choice, [midwifery] has been more and more a profession" like obstetrics.

The unlicensed midwives know that licensure will probably dictate whom they can accept as clients, what procedures they may use, and when they must transfer a client or newborn for medical care. They fear that the screening criteria and transfer regulations will reflect physicians' pathological view of childbirth and take away many of their clients. They worry especially that licensure may prevent them from suturing tears and from administering drugs and setting up IVs in the case of hemorrhages. Most believe that such limitations would make their practices irresponsible.

The unlicensed midwives feel that unreasonable restrictions are more likely to occur if physicians and nurses control the regulatory board. For this reason, many qualify their support of licensure to include only a system in which lay midwives control, or at least are adequately represented on, the board.

In spite of their concerns, most unlicensed midwives will accept restrictions on their practice in return for legality and the better relations with physicians which they expect will follow. Only two express doubts about whether these expectations are realistic. One of these says:

> Even if [midwives] were recognized legally, I think the respect would be hard to come by. . . . This doctor . . . who was always making these ridiculous put-down statements, I don't think it would stop if people were licensed. I think there would still be certain kinds of harassment.

REALITIES

Restrictions on Clientele and Requirements for Consultation

Licensure laws limit midwives to attend low risk, normal births. The definition of what constitutes a low risk, normal birth is, however, subject to interpretation. Some public health authorities view any kind of chemical or instrumental intervention as abnormal, including using drugs to augment slow labors, cutting episiotomies, and suturing tears. Others consider these typical obstetrical procedures normal and limit their definition of abnormal to inductions, forceps or vacuum extractions, and cesarean sections. The definition of low risk status is subject to even greater debate, with some physicians denying the very existence of such a category. Controversy over the definition of low risk, normal births has produced the observed variations in the degree of restrictiveness of state licensure laws. Nevertheless, on the whole these laws are remarkably similar with respect to screening criteria and practice guidelines. The more liberal laws, such as that in New Mexico, differ only in officially allowing midwives to cut emergency episiotomies and to suture small tears and administer antihemorrhagic drugs with physician approval.

Arizona has one of the more restrictive licensure laws. Licensed midwives in that state may not accept women considered at high risk for a variety of reasons, such as a previous cesarean section or suspected twins.[1] Numerous other conditions require a midwife to consult with a physician before accepting a woman as a client.[2]

Licensed midwives' clients are required to have a third trimester examination supervised by a physician, the standard obstetric laboratory tests of blood and urine, and a formal arrangement for medical backup. The midwives must consult a woman's backup physician if any abnormality develops that changes her risk status. While the law specifies some of these potential complications, Practice Guidelines, issued by the Advisory Committee, elaborate on the rules and make additional recommendations designed to establish a higher standard of care.[3]

Not all the conditions requiring consultation result in terminating midwifery care. Some (such as varicosities or high newborn weight)

1. Other prohibited categories include women under 15 or those with marked skeletal abnormalities, chronic or acute medical conditions such as diabetes or active herpes, severe mental retardation, drug addiction, alcohol consumption in excess of two ounces per day, or those with a fetal anomaly that may require immediate medical management after delivery. Neither may they accept women as clients whose planned location for delivery is unsafe due to lack of cleanliness or a telephone, who are unwilling to accept the midwife's legal limitations, or who lack backup medical care.

2. These include more than four previous births, age 15 to 18 or over 35, and a history of a maternal or newborn complication such as premature labors or perinatal loss.

3. These recommendations include a physician visit early in pregnancy, the standard obstetrical schedule for prenatal visits, assessments to make during the pregnancy and childbirth, a postpartum stay longer than the 2 hours required by law, a newborn examination by a pediatrician in the first few days after birth, and two follow-up postpartum visits in addition to the one required in the first 72 hours.

rarely do, whereas others (such as fetal death, premature onset of labor, breech presentation, fetal distress, postpartum hemorrhage, laceration repair, or newborn respiratory distress) always do. In other cases, the decision to terminate or transport lies with the consulting physician. Examples of these discretionary cases include women who have not gone into labor by 42 weeks gestation, those whose duration of labor has gone beyond the norms generally accepted by physicians, and newborns with abnormal color. In many cases, the licensed midwives resume care after physicians have dealt with the complications. The most common example is the resumption of postpartum care after a physician or certified nurse-midwife has sutured a laceration.

In contrast to the unlicensed midwives' fears that licensure would restrict their clientele, few of the licensed midwives feel hampered by their required screening criteria. Many have added additional criteria of their own such as not attending women who smoke or who drink alcohol during pregnancy. As mentioned in chapter 3, the most common nonmedical reason why midwives decline to accept a client or terminate care is a feeling that the woman is irresponsible in her diet, exercise, sleep pattern, or general behavior. These self-imposed restrictions derive from lay midwives' holistic, wellness orientation and their emphasis on personal responsibility for health.

The maternity care philosophy of unlicensed midwives does not differ from that of licensed midwives. Although both groups stress the desirability of individualized care, however, only unlicensed midwives can use this belief as a basis for flexibility in their acceptance criteria for clients. All unlicensed midwives currently use more liberal guidelines, particularly in regard to age and previous history of maternal or newborn complications, than allowed in most states that license lay midwives. Nevertheless, the difference in clientele is not as great as one might expect. In most cases, Arizona's licensed midwives may attend such women if they can obtain physician approval. Other kinds of cases involving overt prohibitions under Arizona's law such as breeches, premature babies, twins, or women who previously have had cesareans are attended by very few of the unlicensed midwives. One of those previously willing to attend these higher risk cases now tries to convince such women to go to a hospital because of "political" concerns about medical opinion of midwives.

Arizona's licensed midwives also have no quarrel with most of the required and recommended reasons for medical consultations. Their philosophy of individualized care, however, leads many to express skepticism that, if a client does not follow the medical profession's time norms for each stage of labor, she is necessarily abnormal and high risk. If a client is making slow but observable progress toward a delivery and wants to remain at home, and no fetal difficulties are indicated, most licensed midwives feel that they should be allowed to continue attending the client. Obtaining a physician's approval to do so depends largely on whether the client has a backup arrangement with a supportive physician. This is not always the case. In some areas of the state no physician will provide personal backup. In these instances, midwives must rely on public hospitals where obstetrical staff members will not take responsibility for an unfamiliar midwife's client without physically evaluating her. The antepartum transfer rate is substantially higher in these areas.

None of the unlicensed midwives believes that the accepted medical time norms for labor and delivery accurately indicate the need to consult a physician. The lack of constraint on unlicensed midwives produces a significant difference in their rate of transfer to medical care compared to Arizona's licensed midwives. Whereas prolonged labor is the most common reason for predelivery hospital transport of licensed midwives' clients (see chap. 6 for more details), most unlicensed midwives report that they seldom transfer for this reason.

Restrictions on Clinical Practices

Although Arizona's licensed midwives have relatively few complaints about client screening and medical consultation regulations, most feel strongly that the restrictions on clinical practices keep "one of our hands tied behind our back" and deny the home birth woman "the same opportunities for emergency care available to hospital patients." These restrictions, in effect at the time of the interviews, prohibit episiotomies, the use of antihemorrhagic drugs (including herbs) and IVs, and the suturing of lacerations. The midwives want the right to use these interventionist techniques, but they want them restricted to emergency situations. They recognize that physicians over time incorporated various procedures initially developed for emergency use into the routine management of childbirth. Fear that a similar routinization of emergency procedures might occur among midwives led three licensed midwives to argue against expanding their own rights to perform such procedures. The others, along with their association, have lobbied extensively for loosening these restrictions.

The concern that liberalizing licensure prohibitions will lead to overuse of interventions is not supported by the evidence from unlicensed midwives. All the unlicensed midwives say that they would cut an emergency episiotomy, yet they regard this intervention as undesirable except in rare emergencies involving fetal distress. Many have never done one. The three most experienced midwives have done a total of six episiotomies during the approximately 700 births they have attended in total.

In contrast, suturing is far more common among unlicensed midwives. Three-quarters of them say that they suture most small lacerations, and the rest always work with a partner who does repairs. All report transferring women with more extensive lacerations to medical care. Most states that license midwives allow them to suture and there have been no reports of abuse of this procedure.

Allowing midwives to use drugs carries a far greater potential for abuse. Some of the licensed midwives and 86 percent of the unlicensed midwives admit that they carry illegal antihemorrhagic medications for emergency use. These same drugs can be used to stimulate contractions during labor, although none says that she uses them for this reason. Some unlicensed midwives, however, carry herbs to augment slow labors and to use as a first attempt to control hemorrhages. Others in their state view herbs as drugs of unknown potency and danger and question their use by midwives.

The use of any chemical for active management of labor is unlikely to be common since it conflicts with the midwives' advocacy of passive management. No Arizona midwife expresses a desire to use drugs to augment labor, and only one wants access to drugs for pain relief. The extent to which drugs are or would be used to control hemorrhages is more difficult to assess. All midwives, licensed and unlicensed, fear maternal hemorrhages and most worry that relying only on manual control could compromise a client. Most states that license midwives, other than Arizona, allow them to administer an emergency antihemorrhagic. No reports have appeared citing abuse of this privilege. For unlicensed midwives the use of antihemorrhagics is undoubtedly tempered by their fear of legal repercussions. As one says:

It is sometimes really gut-wrenching to put yourself in situations where you know that you have to use this for this woman's health and safety and whatever. But when we transfer her, I may really be putting myself in a terrible position here. . . . If I have someone hemorrhaging and I give them the drug, I know that, if we have to go to the nearest hospital, I'm going to have to tell them that she has had xxx. That is hard.

Although the decision to use an illegal drug may be difficult, it was clear from the interviews that the majority of unlicensed midwives will do so when it appears necessary.

Medical Control and Supervision
Another issue raised by unlicensed midwives is the likelihood that licensure would place them under the supervision and control of medical practitioners. They point to the constraining effect that this has had on certified nurse-midwives who are either legally prohibited from attending home births or who cannot find a physician willing to supervise them in home births or free-standing birth centers. The majority, who do not want to become certified nurse-midwives, also feel that certified nurse-midwives' training and certification requirements socialize them to accept the medical, disease-oriented view of pregnancy and childbirth.

The unlicensed midwives believe that licensed midwives' training and examinations have a similar medicalizing influence. In Arizona, however, all past training programs have been run by lay or licensed midwives independent of hospitals, unlike certified nurse-midwifery programs. These programs have relied on current obstetrical literature no more heavily than the proprietary midwifery course in the northeastern state.

The role of required training is probably less important for exposing midwives to the medical model than is the nature of the licensure examination. In Arizona, the examinations in the first six years of the reactivated program were largely written by the program's nurse-midwife directors, subject to Advisory Board approval. A licensed midwife now oversees the program, but her examinations still must pass the scrutiny of the Advisory Board. This board always has been chaired by a perinatologist and has contained one or two other physicians. One of these physicians is usually a neonatalogist; if not, a nurse-neonatologist is appointed. Although this structure assures medical control, midwives have considerable influence through their three representatives on the board. The other members of the board include a consumer and a certified nurse-midwife.

Over the years, a few prospective midwives have complained that the examinations have contained too many questions on pathological problems, medical theory, and medical interventions rather than focusing on the proper care of normal childbirth and the recognition of problems requiring medical assistance. The certified nurse-midwife in charge of revising the 1982 examination concluded that 6 percent of the objective questions covered rare complications or theory outside of midwives' parameters and not essential for safe practice. Surprisingly few of the licensed midwives object to such questions. More recent examinations have included fewer of these kinds of questions and more questions on recognition of early signs of potential problems (such as unusually high weight gain that might foretell pre-eclampsia and require careful monitoring). The more recent examinations also contain an essay section on managing complications.

Licensure also increases midwives' exposure to the medical model through continuing education programs run by physicians and certified nurse-midwives, on topics such as newborn resuscitation and management of maternal hemorrhage. The midwives have organized some of these programs to meet perceived training needs, and the state has encouraged them to attend other programs planned for physicians and certified nurse-midwives.

Through the examination process and the establishment of practice guidelines and educational requirements, regulatory boards act as the gatekeepers and standard setters of licensed midwifery. In Arizona midwives are well-represented on their board and have few complaints about its composition. Although the presence of nonmidwives makes it a form of external regulation, unlike the self-regulating medical boards or the trade associations of unlicensed midwives, the substantial number of midwife representatives makes it a relatively mild form of medical control. Similar situations prevail in other states with licensing, such as South Carolina, New Mexico, and Washington.

The extent to which licensed midwives are directly controlled by physicians depends on the structure of each state's licensure law. Arizona's law specifically acknowledges licensed midwives as independent practitioners, not required to practice under physician supervision. On the surface this would seem ideal from the midwives' perspective, but the state's requirements for medical screening and backup of clients makes the midwives ultimately dependent on physicians. In this respect the introduction of licensure has not changed the nature of the midwife-physician relationship; unlicensed midwives also must depend on physician cooperation to practice in a way they feel is safe and appropriate.

Pressures toward Hierarchical Relationships
Licensure has, however, contributed indirectly to changes in the relationship between midwives and clients. As chapter 3 describes, the midwives strongly believe in sharing responsibility and decision-making with their clients. For licensed midwives, awareness of their legal responsibilities now tempers this ideological commitment. If they do not follow the state's guidelines, they risk losing their licenses and livelihoods. Moreover, as licensed practitioners their work is open to scrutiny by the public, the state, and the medical profession, leaving them little leeway to follow clients' desires, should those desires fall too far outside accepted protocols. As a result, all except one of the licensed midwives report that they would override clients' decisions or terminate care before jeopardizing either client safety or their own licenses. Most require clients to sign an agreement acknowledging that the midwife must work within the state's guidelines and has final say regarding the need for medical consultation or care.

Licensure also has fostered a more hierarchical style of practice by facilitating changes in midwives' clientele. To the extent that licensure has increased midwifery's visibility, accessibility, and acceptability, it has encouraged a broadening of midwives' clientele beyond those who share midwives' philosophy of childbirth. Many now choose midwifery care simply as the cheapest option. These individuals expect and pressure midwives to control their care much as a physician would.

EVALUATING THE EFFECTS OF LICENSURE

In a recent article (1986), DeVries has argued that licensure will destroy lay midwifery and that only "those who stay outside the law . . . have the benefit of remaining true to their own ideals of practice" (1986:1147). He asserts that licensure

> typically places midwives under the control of boards dominated by physicians and nurses. Licensure requires midwives to take examinations created by physicians, covering knowledge developed by physicians about the birth process. Such examinations rarely test knowledge of non-interventive techniques and other styles of care derived from the tradition of midwifery. Licensure requires training in state-approved programs created and usually approved by physicians. [As a result,] the licensing process . . . is certain to diminish the alternative character of the profession in time. (1148–49)

In a previous publication (1985:89–117), DeVries additionally claims that licensure subverts midwifery by restricting practice to those who can afford lengthy training, restricting clients to those defined as low risk by physicians and restricting techniques to those considered safe by medical superiors. Finally, he avers that licensure diminishes the uniqueness of midwifery by encouraging individuals to enter the field simply to earn a living rather than out of commitment to its original philosophy. He fears that such midwives are likely to build bigger practices, sacrifice individualized and holistic care, and eventually succumb to the temptation of a hospital-based practice.

DeVries bases these conclusions largely on a comparison of the fates of certified nurse-midwives and unlicensed midwives. Yet these groups are not comparable. As we have described in chapter 1, certified nurse-midwifery grew out of nursing and has remained a subordinated field under the direct control of supervising physicians. Contemporary lay midwifery, in contrast, developed outside the medical hierarchy as a consumer-based response to the excesses of modern medicine. That most certified nurse-midwives trained and working in hospitals continue to have a more medicalized philosophy and practice tells us much about the contextual effect of the hospital but nothing about the impact of licensing laws.

Our data comparing licensed and unlicensed midwives suggest that licensure is only one of many factors eroding the unique qualities of lay midwifery. As middle-class citizens of a highly medicalized society, both licensed and unlicensed midwives seek access to medical literature. Left to their own resources, the self-imposed training reg-

imen of unlicensed midwives is remarkably similar to that of midwives working under a licensing system. Other changes that DeVries
attributes to licensure also have emerged in its absence. With increased knowledge and experience, both licensed and unlicensed
midwives have moderated some of their earlier beliefs and practices
in quite similar ways, as chapter 8 will discuss. Many of the other
changes DeVries notes are the results of midwifery's success. While
licensure has contributed to midwifery's visibility, accessibility, and
acceptability, similar developments have occurred in states without
licensure laws, although not to the same extent. It is this natural
growth—facilitated by but not dependent on licensure—that has
changed the nature of midwifery's clientele and encouraged midwives to enlarge their practices, thus reducing to a small degree their
ability to provide holistic, individualized, nonhierarchical care.

Finally, midwives have proved susceptible to medicalization because they rely on medicine for most of their knowledge base. Unlike
chiropractors or acupuncturists, they have no alternative theory of
childbirth physiology that stands independent of medicine. For this
reason, they always have seen themselves as part of the continuum of
care rather than as a complete alternative to the medical mainstream.
The subtle changes that we have documented in midwifery reflect
the natural history of any growing occupation rather than solely the
results of licensure.

REFERENCES

Anisef, Paul, and Priscilla Basson. "The institutionalization of a profession: A
    comparison of British and American midwifery." *Sociology of Work and
    Occupation* 6:353–72, 1979.
DeVries, Raymond G. "The contest for control: Regulating new and expand-
    ing health occupations." *American Journal of Public Health* 76:1147–50,
    1986.
DeVries, Raymond G. *Regulating Birth: Midwives, Medicine, and the Law.* Phila-
    delphia: Temple University Press, 1985.
Devitt, Neal. "The statistical case for elimination of the midwife: Fact versus
    prejudice, 1890–1935" (Part 2). *Women and Health* 4:169–86. Summer
    1979.
MANA News. "Interim registry board to refine latest proposal." 4:2, 1987.
Shaw, George B. *The Doctor's Dilemma.* London: Constable, 1930.

CHAPTER 6
THE QUESTION OF RISK

State legislatures that have outlawed lay midwifery have done so on the assumption that a home birth, especially if attended by a nonphysician, is unsafe. Echoing the vehement opposition of physicians, they argue that any increased physical risk for mothers and babies supercedes constitutional guarantees of free trade and self-determination. The issue of safety is paramount in the minds of midwives as well. As previous chapters have discussed, many decide to attend home births because they believe that standard hospital obstetrical practices create undue hazards for normal childbirth. They believe that midwife-attended home birth is a safe alternative for low risk women.

The question of relative risks is not easily resolved. The review of existing research presented in this chapter reveals that most previous studies of home birth outcomes suffer from serious methodological problems. All these studies, including the new data presented in this chapter, can be criticized for examining only the immediate, rather than long-term, physical outcomes of midwife-attended home births. Also, detailed information is not available on the outcomes of all cases transferred prior to delivery because some hospitals exclude midwives from labor and delivery rooms and hospitals do not make their records available to midwives. Moreover, no study can accurately compare home birth outcomes with hospital outcomes unless based on a randomized experimental design and none has been done.

In the absence of a more rigorous experimental design, comparisons between hospital and midwife-attended home birth outcomes are of limited value. Differences in outcomes are confounded with differences in the relative risk statuses of the populations served. All home birth midwives screen potential clients and refer those that they consider too risky to physicians for hospital delivery. Clients who develop problems during labor also are transferred to physicians for hospital delivery. Although some midwives use more stringent criteria for screening and transfer than others, midwives' home birth clients as a group have a lower risk profile than that of women attended in hospital by physicians.

PREVIOUS RESEARCH

The American College of Obstetricians and Gynecologists (1978) has publicized vital statistic data showing higher perinatal mortality among out-of-hospital births than hospital births as proof that home birth is dangerous. A more detailed analysis of one state's vital statistics, published in the *American Journal of Obstetrics and Gynecology* (Shy et al., 1980), also is cited frequently by physicians in support of their opposition to home birth. Vital statistic data, however, do not distinguish between planned and unplanned out-of-hospital births. Researchers in North Carolina and Kentucky find that 22 and 29 percent, respectively, of out-of-hospital births in these states are unplanned (Burnett et al., 1980; Hinds et al., 1985). The majority of these unplanned births are precipitous and have almost a seven-fold increased risk of low birth weight compared with planned out-of-hospital births (Hinds et al., 1985). Given the strong relationship between low birth weight and perinantal mortality (McCormick, 1985; Taffel, 1986), these unplanned home births have a major impact on the overall perinatal mortality of out-of-hospital births. As a result, aggregate out-of-hospital birth outcomes cannot be used as a proxy for planned home birth outcomes.

Several studies of vital statistical data have attempted to distinguish planned from unplanned out-of-hospital births by type of attendant (Clark and Bennetts, 1982; Dingley, 1979), type of attendant and weight of newborn (Burnett et al., 1980), follow-up interviews (Cameron et al., 1979), and mailed questionnaires (Hinds et al., 1985). In each case the researchers find no evidence that planned out-of-hospital birth is associated with an increased risk of neonatal death. Instead, they find a lower incidence of neonatal mortality and low birth weight babies among planned out-of-hospital births in spite of, in at least one state (Burnett et al., 1980), a higher risk demographic profile among the mothers.

Such favorable findings must be regarded with caution. As the authors of these studies note, home birth mothers have lower medical risks than hospital birth mothers for the reasons discussed in the introduction to this chapter. In addition, neonatal mortality and birth weight, although extremely important, do not capture the full range of potential morbidity among newborns; the possibility of subsequent developmental problems due to unnoticed oxygen deprivation cannot be ruled out with vital statistical data. The rarity of neonatal deaths among planned, out-of-hospital births further undermines the validity of these favorable findings. Since out-of-hospital births, though increasing, still account for fewer than 5 percent of births in the states considered and since neonatal deaths are also rare events, an outcome study focused on neonatal mortality needs an extremely large number of cases to find statistically significant relationships. The Kentucky study, for example, included only 465 planned home births and there were no neonatal deaths among them (Hinds et al., 1985). The largest number of planned, midwife-attended, out-of-hospital births in these studies is 1,597 Oregon births, which resulted in only five neonatal deaths (Clark and Bennetts, 1982).

In lieu of larger numbers, some researchers using vital statistical data have tried to identify deaths that might have been prevented if the women had delivered in, rather than out of, hospitals. These cases are often highly conjectural, especially when parents' plans for home or hospital births are not identified. Shy and associates (1980), for example, suggest that some cases of neonatal death due to prematurity and two cases of early neonatal homicide might have been averted if the births had taken place in a hospital. However, the deaths from prematurity are far more likely to have been planned hospital deliveries interrupted by precipitous onset of labor than planned home births. Similarly, the fact that homicides have occurred tells us nothing about the inherent risks of home birth, since there are no grounds for assuming that hospitals could have prevented these tragedies. Rather, the holistic care offered by home birth midwives would have been more likely than medical care to uncover and resolve any serious emotional problems. In the North Carolina study, which distinguishes planned from unplanned out-of-hospital births, all three of the midwife-attended out-of-hospital deaths were due to congenital anomalies (Burnett et al., 1980:2743). In contrast, 77 percent of the deaths among unplanned out-of-hospital births followed precipitous deliveries and 17 percent were suspected homicide or neglect. In the Oregon study, one of the five midwife-attended neonatal deaths was due to congenital anomalies, one had low birth weight, one was attributed to perinatal conditions, and two were labeled sudden infant death syndrome (Clarke and Bennetts, 1982).

The Oregon study (Clark and Bennetts, 1982) is hampered by inappropriate comparisons among birth attendants. The researchers grouped physicians, naturopaths, chiropractors, nurses, and emergency medical personnel in one category of attendants and certified nurse-midwives and lay midwives in another. More generally, none of the outcome studies using data from vital statistics controls for quality of training among lay midwives.

A study by Mehl and associates (1977) was designed to circumvent the fact that vital statistics identify neither out-of-hospital birth attendants' skills nor planned delivery location, as well as the problems of comparing home and hospital birth outcomes. That study compares the medical records on 1,146 planned home births from five selected home delivery services. The five services chosen include three staffed by physicians and nurse assistants and two staffed only by lay midwives. The data provide a comparison of the outcomes of planned home births supervised by physicians with those supervised by lay midwives whom the researchers judged to be competent. Although the lay midwives are self-taught, unlicensed, and unregulated, the rates of complications and perinatal mortality in all five services are similar. They also are lower than the state average, as one would expect given a lower risk clientele. Moreover, the Apgar scores, which measure newborn condition, were higher, a finding which the authors attribute to the absence of pain-relief drugs in the out-of-hospital setting.

These results must be considered with caution. While the risk status of the lay midwives' home birth clientele resembles that of the physicians' home birth clientele more than that of hospital maternity

patients, the risk statuses of the physicians' and lay midwives' populations do differ. A higher proportion of the lay midwives' clients later
decided against home birth, and the lay midwives did not knowingly
attend breech or twin deliveries whereas the physicians sometimes
did. Also, the lay midwives transferred all cases of arrested labor and
more cases of prolonged rupture of membranes to the hospital than
did physicians who could use oxytocin to stimulate labor.

In a subsequent study designed to overcome the limitations of their
earlier studies, Mehl and associates (1980) retrospectively compare
midwife-attended planned home births with a sample of physician-
attended planned hospital births. Cases were matched for maternal
age, education, parity, length of gestation, presentation, and risk
score. There are no significant differences in birth weight, perinatal
mortality, or other major complications. However, compared to the
matched hospital cases, the home birth cases are characterized by
higher Apgar scores and significantly less fetal distress, meconium
staining, postpartum hemorrhage, birth injuries, and need for infant
resuscitation.

The evidence from these two studies strongly suggests that home
delivery can be a safe alternative for medically screened, healthy
women if attended by physicians or selected, experienced midwives.
However, the authors' retrospective analysis is limited by the debatable completeness and accuracy of the records which they reviewed
and the lack of matches for atypical women. Even more important,
the researchers may have biased the outcome data in favor of midwives by including only those midwives whom they judged to be
competent. They acknowledge that there are "ample numbers of
anecdotes about women who have seen one or two births and then
called themselves midwives" (1980:20). This, in fact, is exactly how
some of the lay midwives that they selected for their first study started
out (1977:282).

LICENSED MIDWIVES' CLIENTS

States which license and actively monitor the practice of lay midwifery offer researchers the advantage of a registry of planned home
births and records of their outcomes. In addition, all licensed midwives have met established criteria for practice, eliminating the possi-

ble selectivity bias of other studies. This section adds four years of data to a previous analysis of planned home birth outcomes during the first four years of Arizona's reactivated licensed midwifery program (Sullivan and Beeman, 1983). During these eight years, licensed midwives attended 3,666 labors, resulting in 3,255 out-of-hospital births. The vast majority of these births occurred in private homes, although a few of the midwives with high volume practices have established clinics in their own homes or on commercial property.

The state's laws for midwifery practice are designed to limit licensed midwives to low risk clients, as chapter 5 explains. As a result, very few of their clients have problematic obstetrical histories, and most are in the optimum age range for childbearing (table 6.1). More than two-thirds previously had given birth and only three percent had five or more births.

The primary responsibility of midwives under the state's laws is to look for changes in risk status. All require their clients to see them on a regular basis for prenatal care; 85 percent of the clients had 5 or more prenatal visits and 46 had more than 10. Many urge their clients to have routine medical prenatal care in addition to their midwifery prenatal care. As a result, some clients have far more prenatal medical visits than the single, required, third trimester evaluation. Data collected since 1980 indicate that 27 percent had 4 or more medical visits. The majority of these visits are routine and simply verify that risk status has not changed. When midwives suspect that a problem may be developing, they must have their client consult a physician. However, not all these consults result in a termination. In 1984, for example, 26 women whom midwives transported to physicians for urinary tract infections, varicosities, suspected postmaturity, low fetal heart tones, abnormal fetal growth patterns, traces of meconium, and prolonged rupture of membranes were approved for continued midwifery care and home birth.

TERMINATION OF CARE

Because of the conservative screening, only a small portion of clients accepted for care are subsequently terminated due to medical problems that develop during pregnancy. The Department of Maternal

Table 6.1 Characteristics of 3,972 Midwifery Clients in Arizona, 1978–1985

Characteristics	Attended in Labor 1978–81	Accepted for Care 1982–85
N	1,449	2,523
Maternal Age		
15–19	6%	6%
20–24	37	31
25–29	38	37
30–34	15	20
35–50	4	6
Unknown (32)		
Gravida		
1	20	18
2	34	25
3	22	25
4	12	16
5+	12	16
Unknown (14)		
Parity		
0	33	28
1	34	32

Note: The data for 1982–85 include all cases accepted for care, including those terminated prior to labor. The data for 1978–81 include only those attended in labor because data on terminated cases were not uniformly reported before the 1980s. The Maternal and Child Health Department in

(continued)

and Child Health introduced special forms in 1984 to record information on the reasons for termination. As is evident in table 6.2, some of these terminations are for nonmedical reasons: the client changes her mind about a home birth, decides to use another midwife, or moves away from the area. Only 9 percent of clients accepted for care are terminated for medical problems before a midwife attends their labor. The most common medical reasons are premature onset of labor, rupture of membranes, or delayed onset of labor beyond the 42 weeks gestation allowed in the regulations. These, together with the other medical reasons, reclassify the women as

Table 6.1 (continued)

Characteristics	Attended in Labor 1978–81	Accepted for Care 1982–85
Parity		
2	18	21
3	8	11
4	4	5
5+	4	3
Unknown (9)		
Prenatal Midwife Visits[a]		
Fewer than 5	16	15
5–9	38	39
10–12	31	28
13+	15	18
Unknown (25)		
Prenatal Medical Visits[a]		
1		34
2		31
3–9		32
10+		3
Unknown (142)		

1981 urged midwives to report information on their terminations. A special form was introduced in 1984 to record this information.

[a] The data for 1982–85 include cases terminated from care. As a result midwives do not always report or know the number of prenatal visits eventually made by the client.

higher risk and no longer appropriate for a licensed midwife's services.

TRANSPORT BEFORE BIRTH

Problems can also develop in labor that require a midwife to consult the woman's backup physician and transport her to medical care if directed. Eleven percent of the clients attended in labor by the midwives over the eight years gave birth in a hospital. Most of the indications for transfer, listed in table 6.3, involve changes in risk status, primarily prolonged labor, although clients sometimes request transfer because they want pain relief medication.

MATERNAL OUTCOMES

Maternal outcomes for the 3,255 midwife-assisted births are presented in table 6.4. These aggregate statistics mask several significant improvements that occurred in the first four years of the program (Sullivan and Beeman, 1983). For example, in 1978 only 46 and 38 percent of clients, respectively, had less than one-half hour of second stage of labor and one-quarter hour of third stage compared to 66 and 78 percent, respectively, in 1980. The incidence of second-degree lacerations declined from 22 percent in 1978 to 12 percent in 1979. Blood loss also declined between 1978 and 1979, and again between 1982 and 1983, with only 5 to 6 percent of clients experiencing a loss of 500 or more milliliters in recent years.

Overall, 14 percent of the 3,255 women attended by midwives out-of-hospital were transported for medical care after birth. This aggregate rate also obscures a good deal of change over the time period. As is evident in table 6.5, the most common reason for a postpartum transport is a second-degree laceration. As discussed above, such lacerations declined dramatically between the first and second years

Table 6.2 Reasons for Termination of Midwifery Care in Arizona, 1985

	Number	Percent
Clients Accepted for Care	774	100
Clients Terminated from Care	123	16
Nonmedical Reasons	50	6
Medical Reasons	73	9
Elevated blood pressure (pre-eclampsia)	7	
Bleeding in third trimester	3	
Premature rupture of membranes/labor	9	
Multiple gestation	5	
Problems with fetus: growth, activity, heart rate	6	
Presentation not vertex	3	
42 weeks gestation	13	
Other medical problems	27	

Table 6.3 Indications for Transfer during 3,666 Labors Attended by Arizona
Midwives That Resulted in Hospital Deliveries, 1978–1985

Indications	Number
Clients Attended in Labor	3,666
Labor Complications	
Premature labor	28
Prolonged first stage	136
Prolonged second stage	44
Prolonged rupture of membranes	50
Maternal Indications	
Elevated blood pressure	17
Bleeding	20
Elevated temperature	1
Fetal Indications	
Meconium staining	43
Fetal distress (low, high, or irregular fetal heart rate)	42
Malpresentation	
Unengaged head	29
Not vertex	30
Other (including nonmedical)[a]	76
Clients admitted to hospital for birth (11%)	411

Note: The indications for transfer are not mutually exclusive due to
women with multiple indications, including conditions leading to previous
consults in which physicians approved continued care.
[a] Includes 42 weeks gestation, varicosities, decreased fetal activity, multiple
gestation, and desire for pain relief.

of the program. Some midwives also have made arrangements in the
last few years with physicians or certified nurse-midwives to repair
lacerations at the home or birth clinic. Combined with the decline in
the proportion of clients with heavy blood loss, these changes resulted in a substantial reduction in the postpartum transfer rate from
26 percent in 1978 to 10 percent in the last four years.

Because laceration repair is the major reason for postpartum
transport, only 14 percent of the women transported for medical
care after an out-of-hospital birth were hospitalized. These postpartum hospitalizations constituted a mere 2 percent of all women at-

Table 6.4 Maternal Outcomes of 3,255 Midwife-Assisted Out-of-Hospital Births in Arizona, 1978–1985

	Percent		Percent
First Stage		Estimated Blood Loss	
Less than 9 hours	73	Less than 500 ml	92
9–13 hours	16	500–999 ml	7
13–19 hours	7	1,000+ ml	1
19+ hours	3	Lacerations[a]	
Second Stage		First degree[b]	4
Less than $\frac{1}{2}$ hour	65	Second degree	11
$\frac{1}{2}$–1 hour	21	Third degree	1
1–1$\frac{1}{2}$ hours	7	Fourth degree	...
1$\frac{1}{2}$–2 hours	4	Periurethral	...
2+ hours	3		
Third Stage			
Less than $\frac{1}{4}$ hour	70		
$\frac{1}{4}$–$\frac{1}{2}$ hour	23		
$\frac{1}{2}$–$\frac{3}{4}$ hour	5		
$\frac{3}{4}$–1 hour	1		
1+ hours	1		

[a] Some of the women with lacerations were not transported because a physician or certified nurse-midwife came to the house to repair the laceration or because the laceration was not judged to need surgical repair.

[b] First-degree lacerations are underreported because the vast majority of cases do not require medical care.

tended out-of-hospital by midwives. Like the overall transfer rate, the rate of postpartum hospitalization following a midwife-attended birth has declined over the period; the rate in the last four years has been 1 percent compared with not quite 3 percent in the first four years. This reduction is associated with the decreased rate of transfer for postpartum hemorrhage.

NEWBORN OUTCOMES

As a result of both the midwives' conservative screening of prospective clients and emphasis on good nutrition for adequate maternal weight gain, only 1 percent of the 3,257 newborns delivered by the

Table 6.5 Indications for Maternal Transfer after Out-of-Hospital Birth among 3,255 Midwifery Clients in Arizona, 1978–1985

Maternal Complications after Home Birth	Number
Labor Problems[a]	78
Postpartum hemorrhage	72
Shock	11
Uterine atony	20
Retained placenta	41
Retained placenta fragments or membranes	24
Elevated temperature	9
Laceration:	
First degree	27
Second degree	267
Third degree	18
Fourth degree	2
Periurethral	2
Other[b]	41
Number of Women Transported after an Out-of-Hospital Birth (14%)	442
Number of Women Admitted to a Hospital after an Out-of-Hospital Birth (2%)	63

Note: The indications for transfer categories are not mutually exclusive due to women with multiple indications.

[a] Includes cases where physicians approved continued care after consultation for such problems as evidence of traces of meconium, exceeding length-of-labor or rupture-of-membranes guidelines, and transitory fetal-heart irregularities.

[b] *Other* includes thrombophlebitis and accompanying a transported baby.

licensed midwives were under 2,500 grams compared to the national rate of 7 percent in 1984 (National Center for Health Statistics, 1986:28). Apgar scores were also high; only 3 percent were scored less than seven at five minutes. As Mehl and associates (1977) suggest, this may be due to the absence of pain relief drugs.

Unlike the maternal transport rate, the transport rate for newborns has remained stable at 5 percent over the eight-year period. The most common complication, listed in table 6.6, was respiratory

Table 6.6 Indications for Newborn Transfer after 3,257 Out-of-Hospital Births in
Arizona, 1978–1985

Newborn Complications after Home Birth	Number
Congenital anomalies[a]	16
Respiratory distress	37
Apgar less than 5 at 1 minute	11
Apgar less than 7 at 5 minutes	23
Postmaturity	4
Meconium stain	24
Jaundice[b]	28
Small for gestational age	4
Large for gestational age	16
Other[c]	46
Number of Newborns Transported to medical care (5%)	171
Number of Newborns Admitted to a Hospital (2%)	71

Notes: The indications for transfer categories are not mutually exclusive
due to newborns with multiple indications. The difference between the
number of home births and the number of home-birth women is due to two
sets of unexpected twins.

[a] Congenital anomalies include bilateral club foot, two cases with spina bifida and hydrocephalus, multiple intestinal obstructions, three cleft palates,
tracheo-esophageal fistula, heart defects, Down's syndrome, trisomy 18,
Turner's syndrome, scalp deformity, diaphragmatic hernia, and oomphalo-
cele.

[b] Found on required postpartum home visits.

[c] *Other* includes ABO incompatability, flushed red, pale, cyanotic, or gray,
abnormal cry, lethargy, poor feeding, abnormal head circumference, no
meconium in 24 hours, abnormal cord, tachypnea, polycythemia, periodic
apnea, hypothermia, edema of the scrotum and penis, persistent fetal cir-
culation, suspected sepsis, and accompanying the mother for medical care.

distress followed by jaundice and meconium staining. Forty percent
of the newborns transported for medical care were hospitalized, resulting in a 2 percent hospitalization rate for all out-of-hospital births
attended by licensed midwives.

Four fetal deaths have occurred among the 3,666 labors attended
by the licensed midwives. The first fetal death occurred during a
breech delivery managed in the home without medical consultation.

The midwife's license was suspended for violation of the rules and regulations. The second fetal death also resulted in the revocation of a midwife's license because she falsely reported fetal heart tones in her labor records in order to allow her client to deliver a stillborn at home in violation of the state's regulations. The causes of the other two fetal deaths are unknown. In both cases fetal hearts were heard by the midwives late in the second stage. Attempts to resuscitate the stillborns failed. A fifth fetal death occurred when a midwife's client went into labor after 42 weeks gestation. Several days prior to the onset of labor, the client had a reactive nonstress test which indicated that the fetus was not at risk. The client called the midwife early in labor and reported possible meconium. The midwife sent her directly to the hospital, where an external monitor showed good fetal heart tones for the initial 20 minutes but not after she used the restroom. The cause of death was attributed to cord entanglement.

Some additional fetal deaths have occurred after complications during pregnancy which have resulted in termination of midwifery care. For example, in 1985 three women were sent to their physicians because they reported decreased fetal activity, two at 32 weeks gestation and one at 35 weeks. Two of the fetal deaths were attributed to cord entanglement and the other cause of death was unknown. Another client was sent to her physician because of an abnormal fetal growth pattern. The subsequent hospital stillbirth was related to a congenital anomaly.

Three neonatal deaths have occurred among the 3,257 deliveries attended by the licensed midwives during the eight years. All were due to congenital anomalies: one involved heart and lung anomalies, another heart and liver anomalies, and the third died of a congenital diaphragmatic hernia. A fourth neonatal death occurred following a transport to hospital during labor for fetal distress. No cause of death was determined. A fifth neonatal death occurred to a woman terminated from midwifery care because she went into labor at 25 weeks gestation. The severely premature infant expired shortly after birth in the hospital. There has been one reported postneonatal death at three months due to trisomy 18, a genetic disorder. It is possible that other postneonatal deaths have not been reported either because the midwives do not know of them or because the reasons for death were unrelated to prenatal development or childbirth.

The perinatal mortality rate for all labors attended by Arizona's licensed midwives was 2.2 per thousand with a neonatal rate of 1.1 per thousand. This neonatal rate is substantially lower than the 4.6 per thousand reported for the nearly 4,000 low risk labors begun in eleven free-standing birth centers between 1972 and 1979 (Bennetts and Lubic, 1982). The certified nurse-midwives and physicians working in these birth centers may use less conservative screening criteria than the licensed lay midwives. They also use more interventionistic practices; the authors report that 40 percent of cases received analgesia, anaesthesia, sedatives, hypnotics, or tranquilizers, and 5 percent were assisted with forceps or vacuum extraction. A study at a leading medical teaching hospital reported a perinatal death rate of 2.6 per thousand with a neonatal rate of .7 per thousand for normally formed term infants (Stubblefield and Berek, 1980). Deleting the three neonatal deaths due to congenital anomalies yields comparable rates of 1.4 and .3 per thousand, respectively, for the midwife-attended out-of-hospital labors. Although this comparison does not control for risk status of the two populations, it does suggest that there is little, if any, additional risk involved in choosing midwife-attended out-of-hospital birth in Arizona.

THE ETHICS OF CHOOSING ALTERNATIVES

Despite the low mortality rate for midwife-attended births in Arizona, individuals who choose home birth and the midwives who assist them frequently find themselves confronted by physicians, friends, and family who question their ethics, as well as their motives and sanity (Hoff and Schneiderman, 1985). Persons who consider home birth dangerous wonder whether couples should have the right to choose, and midwives the right to provide, this alternative to normative medical practice.

The ethical questions raised by home birth parallel those embedded in discussions of other alternatives to mainstream medical care. In large part, the debate hinges on the question of risk. If it could be proved to everyone's satisfaction that a given alternative were equal or superior to the standard medical treatment, no one would question its adoption, but insufficient evidence exists to do so. Even where reputable data are available, medical prejudices foster continuing arguments and demands for more rigorous analysis. As we have seen with home birth, physicians may present inappropriate evidence to bolster their opposition or may choose to ignore evidence that contradicts their preconceived ideas. The same reaction has been observed with other health care alternatives. Studies demonstrating the effectiveness of acupuncture, for example, have been ignored, since acknowledging its curative properties would force physicians to question some of their basic beliefs about health and illness (Wolpe, 1985).

In the absence of consensus regarding the safety of alternatives, ethical debate focuses on individual rights versus societal obligations (cf. Hegland, 1965; Cantor, 1973; Riga, 1976). The primary principle supporting the choice of alternative treatments, reflected in legal decisions, is the right to bodily integrity and self-determination. Since at least 1914, American courts have upheld the principle that "every human being of adult years and sound mind has a right to determine what shall be done with his own body; and a surgeon who performs an operation without his patient's consent commits an assault" (Schloendorff v. Society of New York Hospital, 1914:93). This idea was incorporated into the American Hospital Association's 1973 "Patient's Bill of Rights" in a clause stating: "The patient has the right to refuse treatment to the extent permitted by law, and to be informed of the medical consequences of his action." The other face of informed consent, it seems, is "informed refusal."

Even when refusal will likely result in death, some ethicists have argued that "it is not medicine's responsibility to prevent tragedies by denying freedom, for that would be the greater tragedy" (Engelhardt, 1975:47). This issue is far from hypothetical. In numerous instances patients have refused treatment for serious illnesses or accidents based on their philosophies regarding what constitutes meaningful and worthwhile life and their right to self-determination (Byrn, 1975; Riga, 1976). In other cases, refusal has been based on religious beliefs, thus raising other first amendment rights (Macklin, 1977:327–29). Jehovah's Witnesses, for example, will reject needed blood transfusions because of their interpretation of the Bible, especially Leviticus 17 (Macklin, 1977:325). They do not believe that God will protect them from death but consider mortal life insignificant compared to eternal life, and they believe that accepting blood transfusions will cost them resurrection and salvation.

Those who support restricting individual self-determination in medical matters argue that the state has the right and the obligation to safeguard its citizens' health. This argument has met with mixed success in the courts in nonreligious cases (Brody, 1981:97) and even less success in religious cases. Physicians have lost most cases involving adult Jehovah's witnesses except when patients appeared mentally incompetent (due to shock or coma) or had dependent children (Macklin, 1977; Byrn, 1975; Paris, 1975). Physicians also have lost most cases involving individuals such as Christian Scientists who avoid medical care altogether, leaving physicians with no legal standing (Macklin, 1977:326).

Legal and ethical authorities and scholars have been considerably more willing to support imposed intervention when the health of a child is at stake (for a review see Shapiro and Barthel, 1986). The doctrine of "parens patriae" grants the state authority to override parental decisions when needed to protect a child's health or welfare (Steinbock, 1984). The courts have unanimously ruled, for example, that Jehovah's Witnesses cannot legally prohibit blood transfusions for their children, on the grounds that religious freedom does not give parents the right to act in ways that will likely result in their children's deaths (Macklin, 1977; Brody, 1981). This principle also explains the state's willingness to force adults to submit to transfusions if they have dependent children to protect children from the traumatic loss of a parent (Nelson et al., 1986:758–59).

Parents' right to reject treatment for their children appears stronger, both legally and ethically, when the quality of the children's increased lifespan is debatable (McCormick, 1974; Engelhardt, 1981; Vitiello, 1986). In a 1983 case involving an infant with spina bifida who required surgery to forestall further brain damage, the U.S. Supreme Court affirmed parents' right to refuse treatment, even when death might result (Weber v. Stony Brook Hospital, 1983). This case generated considerable publicity and horror, particularly within the right-to-life movement. The resulting pressure led Congress to pass the Child Abuse Amendments of 1984, which define withholding treatment from a newborn as child abuse unless treatment would be futile or inhumane. These amendments were overturned by the Supreme Court in 1986 (Bowen v. American Hospital Association, 1986).

Whose interests should prevail—the individual's or the state's—is least clear when a woman's choice will affect her fetus as well as herself. In several cases, physicians have used the law to force women to have fetal surgery, cesarean sections, or blood transfusions, or have tried to enforce standards of conduct believed to protect the fetus, such as restricting drug use (Bowes and Selgestad, 1981; Annas, 1982; Nelson et al., 1986). In these situations, physicians have argued that the interests of the fetus and the mother are antithetical, and that women's individual rights should be limited for the sake of their fetuses.

The doctrine of "parens patriae" gives the state the right to intervene in parental decision-making. As Barbara Rothman points out, if this right is extended to prenatal decisions, pregnant women risk becoming mere "vessels," losing the rights otherwise granted to competent adults (Mackenzie et al., 1986:26). Once women's interests are subsumed under the interests of the fetus, medicine, and the state, ever more stringent legal requirements may be placed on their behavior.

Although parents' rights to refuse treatment for their children or fetuses remain open to question, they retain broad rights to choose alternative treatments. For example, when the parents of a child with Hodgkin's Disease opted on physicians' advice for nontraditional metabolic therapy including laetrile rather than chemotherapy and radiation, they were sued for child neglect (Matter of Hofbauer, 1979). The court dismissed the suit on the grounds that the parents had sought medical advice and assistance and had provided a form of therapy which they believed to be the best "and which has not been totally rejected by all responsible medical authority." This description fits the current position of midwife-attended out-of-hospital births. Although officially rejected by mainstream medical organizations, some responsible medical authorities, including the editor of the leading public health journal (Yankauer, 1983) and faculty from prominent medical schools (for example, Sagov et al., 1984), find it an acceptable alternative.

Underlying these legal and ethical debates is the growth of technological imperialism and medical paternalism (Veatch, 1972). The norms and values of our postindustrial society have created a climate favorable to passive acceptance of new technologies. The mere mechanical ability to do something—whether a medical, military, or industrial technology—often has been sufficient justification for doing it. Yet as chapter 2 has demonstrated, many widely accepted medical treatments adopted in the last 50 years have been found to be dangerous (Mackenzie et al., 1986). Nevertheless, some physicians assume that their technical expertise makes them the most competent persons to determine appropriate medical treatment and limit available alternatives (Veatch, 1972:6).[1] Yet, physicians have no special training or sensitivity which would justify their pivotal role in what are moral as well as medical decisions.

REFERENCES

American College of Obstetricians and Gynecologists. "Health department data shows danger of home births." January 4, 1978.

Annas, George J. "Forced cesareans: The most unkindest cut of all." *Hastings Center Report* 12:16+, 1982.

Bennetts, Anita, and Ruth Lubic. "The free-standing birth centre." *Lancet* 1:378–80, 1982.

Bowen v. American Hospital Association, 106 S. Ct. 2101 (1986).

Bowes, Watson A., and Brad Selgestad. "Fetal versus maternal rights: Medical and legal perspectives." *Obstetrics and Gynecology* 58:209–14, 1983.

Brody, Howard. *Ethical Decisions in Medicine*, 2d ed. Boston: Little, Brown, 1981.

Burnett, Claude, James Jones, Judith Rooks, Chong Hwa Chen, Carl Tyler, and C. Arden Miller. "Home delivery and neonatal mortality in North Carolina." *Journal of the American Medical Association* 244:2741–45, 1980.

Byrn, Robert M. "Compulsory lifesaving treatment for the competent adult." *Fordham Law Review* 44:1–36, 1975.

Cameron, Joyce, Eileen Chase, and Sallie O'Neal. "Home birth in Salt Lake County, Utah." *American Journal of Public Health* 69:716–17, 1979.

Cantor, Norman L. "A patient's decision to decline lifesaving medical treatment: Bodily integrity versus the preservation of life." *Rutgers Law Review* 26:228–64, 1973.

Child Abuse Amendments of 1984, Pub. L. No. 98-457, 98 Stat. 1749 (1984).

Clark, Nancy, and Anita Bennetts. "Vital statistics and nonhospital births: A mortality study of infants born out of hospitals in Oregon," pp. 171–81 (appendix F) in Committee on Assessing Alternative Birth Settings (ed.),

1. For a striking example dealing with conflicting rights of women and fetuses, see Lieberman and Chaim (1979).

Research Issues in the Assessment of Birth Settings. Washington, DC: National Academy Press, 1982.

Dingley, Erma. "Birthplace and attendants: Oregon's alternative experience." *Women and Health* 4:239–53, 1979.

Englehardt, H. Tristram. "A demand to die." *Hastings Center Report* 5:9+, 1975.

Hegland, Kenney F. "Unauthorized rendition of lifesaving medical treatment." *California Law Review* 53:860–77, 1965.

Hinds, M. Ward, Gershon Bergeisen, and David Allen. "Neonatal outcomes in planned v. unplanned out-of-hospital births in Kentucky." *Journal of the American Medical Association* 253:1578–82, 1985.

Hoff, Gerard A., and Lawrence J. Schneiderman. "Having babies at home: Is it safe? Is it ethical?" *Hastings Center Report* 15:19–27, 1985.

Lieberman, J. R., and W. Chaim. "The fetal right to live." *Obstetrics and Gynecology* 53:515–17, 1979.

Mackenzie, Thomas B., Theodore C. Nagel, and Barbara K. Rothman. "When a pregnant woman endangers her fetus." *Hastings Center Report* 16:24–25, 1986.

Macklin, Ruth. "Consent, coercion and conflicts of rights." *Perspectives in Biology and Medicine* 20:360–71, 1977.

Matter of Hofbauer, New York Court of Appeals, 47 N.Y. 2d 648, 419, N.Y. Supp. 2d 936, 1979.

Mehl, Lewis, Gail Peterson, Michael Whitt, and Warren Hawes. "Outcomes of elective home births: A series of 1,146 cases." *Journal of Reproductive Medicine* 19:281–90, 1977.

Mehl, Lewis, Jean-Richard Ramiel, Brenda Leininger, Barbara Hoff, Kathy Kronenthal, and Gail Peterson. "Evaluation of outcomes of non-nurse midwives: Matched comparisons with physicians." *Women and Health* 5:17–29, 1980.

McCormick, Maire. "The contribution of low birth weight to infant mortality and childhood morbidity." *New England Journal of Medicine* 312:82–90, 1985.

National Center for Health Statistics. "Advance report of final natality statistics, 1984." *Monthly Vital Statistics Report* 35, No. 4 DHHS Publication No. (PHS) 86-1120, Public Health Service. Hyattsville, MD: U.S. Government Printing Office, 1986.

Nelson, Lawrence J., Brian P. Buggy, and Carol J. Weil. "Forced medical treatment of pregnant women: 'Compelling each to live as seems good to the rest.'" *Hastings Law Journal* 37:703–64, 1986.

Paris, John J. "Compulsory medical treatment and religious freedom: Whose law shall prevail?" *University of San Francisco Law Review* 10:1–35, 1975.

Riga, Peter J. "Compulsory medical treatment of adults." *Catholic Lawyer* 22:105–37, 1976.

Sagov, Stanley, Richard Feinbloom, and Peggy Spindel. *Home Birth: A Practitioner's Guide to Birth Outside the Hospital.* Rockville, MD: Aspen Systems Corporation, 1984.

Schloendorff v. Society of New York Hospital, 105 N.E. 92 (New York 1914).

Shapiro, Robyn S., and Richard Barthel. "Infant care review committees: An effective approach to the Baby Doe dilemma?" *Hastings Law Journal* 37:827–62, 1986.

Shy, Kirkwood, Floyd Frost, and Jean Ullom. "Out-of-hospital delivery in Washington State, 1975–1977." *American Journal of Obstetrics and Gynecology* 137:547–52, 1980.

Steinbock, Bonnie. "Baby Jane Doe in the courts." *Hastings Center Reports* 14:13–19, 1984.

Stubblefield, Phillip, and Jonathan Berek. "Perinatal mortality in term and post-term births." *Obstetrics and Gynecology* 56:676–82, 1980.

Sullivan, Deborah, and Ruth Beeman. "Four years' experience with home birth by licensed midwives in Arizona." *American Journal of Public Health* 73:641–45, 1983.

Taffel, Selma. "Maternal weight gain and the outcome of pregnancy, United States, 1980." *Vital and Health Statistics Series* 21, No. 44, DHHS Publication No. 86-1922, Public Health Service. Washington, DC: U.S. Government Printing Office, 1986.

Veatch, Robert M. "Models for ethical medicine in a revolutionary age." *Hastings Center Report* 2:5–7, 1972.

Vitiello, Michael. "Baby Jane Doe: Stating a cause of action against the officiores intermeddler." *Hastings Law Journal* 37:863–908, 1986.

Weber v. Stony Brook Hospital, 60 N.Y. 2d 208, 456 N.E. 2d 1186, 469 N.Y.S. 2d 63 (N.Y.), 1983.

Wolpe, Paul R. "The maintenance of professional authority: Acupuncture and the American physician." *Social Problems* 32:409–24, 1985.

Yankauer, Alfred. "The valley of the shadow of birth." *American Journal of Public Health* 73:635–37, 1983.

CHAPTER 7
PHYSICIAN REACTION

The current relationship between midwives and physicians in the United States bears the mark of recent history. The lack of central regulation of midwifery training and standards in the face of the emergent science of obstetrics and the consolidation of physicians' authority led to the granny midwife stereotype discussed in chapter 1. One midwife summarized the common physician view of her predecessors "as a group of dirty, illiterate, alcoholic, old hags that didn't know anything about anything." Like other home birth midwives interviewed, she claims that "the image still persists today." The only difference is that physicians now expect midwives to be more of a "hippie type with long skirts and scarves and beads" who delivers "in a barn in the woods" rather than a Dickensian "Sairey Gamp."

THE MIDWIVES' COMPLAINT

Unlicensed home birth midwives describe the current attitudes of most physicians toward them as "hostile." "Even the supportive ones," they say, "have grave reservations." The midwives cite media coverage of physicians who brand them as "unqualified," "incompetent," "irresponsible," and guilty of "maternal trauma" and "child abuse." The latter two charges were made in an official statement by the former executive director of the American College of Obstetricians and Gynecologists (Obstetrics and Gynecology News, 1977). Although most of these accusations are directed at midwives in general, a few report personal attacks as well. For example, one discussed her frustration when a reporter asked her to respond to the charge, made by the head obstetrician at her local hospital, that she "was constantly bringing in dead babies." She claims that she never has had a death. Without access to hospital records or a regulatory agency monitoring her outcomes, an unlicensed home birth midwife has little credible evidence to counter such accusations.

The licensed midwives report a similar lack of acceptance among most local physicians. They claim that these physicians will not provide private patients with the medical screening and backup required for a home birth. Only a few feel that legalization gives them anything more than begrudged tolerance and reluctant cooperation. They further assert that physicians have used local media to accuse them of delivering breeches and other high risk cases, letting women tear severely and hemorrhage through incompetence, causing mental retardation in newborns by not recognizing oxygen deprivation, and burying stillborns in backyards.

The licensed midwives feel that such accusations amount to a "witch hunt," since state regulation ensures that they maintain high standards of practice. They point to the conservative nature of the state's regulations for screening and practice and the excellent outcomes of their home births, which are a matter of public record (see chap. 6). Moreover, the Bureau of Maternal and Child Health requires detailed reports of every case. These reports, along with any complaints from physicians, are scrutinized for violations of licensure regulations or poor judgment. Despite this constant surveillance, the state has revoked only two midwives' licenses since the program was reactivated—one for complying with parental wishes to deliver a known fetal death at home and the other for not transferring a breech discovered during labor in an isolated area.

In spite of the unanimous claim of widespread physician hostility, most midwives have found one or two physicians to provide medical backup, even though it may mean going to a more distant hospital where the backup has obstetrical privileges. Reported antagonistic incidents such as denying home birth clients medical services, refusing to provide anesthesia when repairing a tear, prohibiting midwives from accompanying their transferred clients into hospitals, and haranguing midwives or their clients for participating in a home birth seem to be confined to a few physicians with extreme views who become the unwilling medical backup in an emergency transfer to a hospital. The more common response of involuntary backup physicians, the midwives say, is to ignore their knowledge of a client's prenatal, labor, and delivery history: "Rather than listen to you . . . they will go ahead and let her labor for another five hours just to see that she's not making progress." However, many midwives report that their clients sometimes receive superior treatment from hospital staff anxious to be accommodating.

The midwives' knowledge of physician hostility comes most often from their clients. When a woman considering a home birth raises the issue with her physician during a prenatal visit, she usually receives a lecture on the risks involved. The midwives claim that most physicians question a midwife's competence and exaggerate the likelihood of problems such as hemorrhages and depressed babies among healthy, nonmedicated, low-risk women. A common claim is that physicians do not regard any women as low risk. The midwives further say that some "rabid" physicians try to scare the women with false stories of dead or severely traumatized mothers and babies brought into the local hospital by midwives.

The midwives attribute physicians' opposition toward them to three causes. The first is concern about the qualifications of both licensed and unlicensed midwives. The second is concern about the risks involved in home birth regardless of the type of attendant. The third is a belief that midwives threaten physicians' medical authority, personal control, and financial monopoly over childbirth.

THE PHYSICIANS' OBJECTIONS

In 1984 we conducted a statewide survey to examine physicians' views of Arizona's midwifery licensure program. All obstetricians and 20 percent of the family and general practitioners received a mail-back questionnaire.[1] A follow-up phone call and second mailing

1. The family or general practitioner sample contains an oversampling of osteopathic physicians to ensure an adequate representation. The sample consisted of 19 percent of the physicians listed as family or general practitioners in the 1983–84 Arizona Medical Directory and 25 percent of those listed in the 1983 Arizona Osteopathic Medical Association Directory. The percentages presented in this chapter have been weighted to compensate for the oversampling of osteopathic general practitioners.

yielded responses from 174 obstetricians (62 percent of the population) and 106 family or general practitioners (51 percent of the sample). The latter group is referred to as general practitioners in the following discussion.

The physicians' responses support the midwives' complaint that most oppose home birth midwives and will not cooperate with the state's midwifery licensure program. General practitioners as well as obstetricians oppose the program, although the latter generally are more strongly opposed and less willing to provide the required screening and medical backup.

The majority of the obstetricians (74 percent) and general practitioners (63 percent) who responded to the survey would like the state to outlaw planned home births by licensed lay midwives. Some indicate that they regard the state's program as regressive, a return to "the dark ages." One adds the comment, "Their patients die! Their babies die! It is medieval 3rd World medicine." Others suggest that it is "the earliest form of child abuse to use untrained and incompetent people for labor and delivery." One writes, "ARIZONA [sic] must protect its desired unborn from McDonald Counter girls who subsidize their income delivering damaged babies." Many others comment that, although they believe in "the patient's right to do whatever she wishes with her own body," they feel that the state "should not endorse and license [midwives] for this purpose." Numerous physicians suggest that licensing "lay" midwives is equivalent to licensing lay lawyers, pilots, engineers, and the like.

Half the obstetricians who responded have received requests from patients to provide medical backup for a licensed-midwife-attended home birth, but only 20 percent of them agreed to help. Even fewer (11 percent) would provide backup if asked by a low-risk patient in the future. A much larger proportion of obstetricians (54 percent) have provided medical care for a home birth midwife's transferred client or newborn as hospital staff or on-call physician. Several comment that they "do not like being placed in this position against [their] will" and that it "usually provides an extremely poor patient-physician relationship under emergency and/or stressful circumstances." One confirms midwives' reports by adding that he has refused to provide care under such circumstances.

General practitioners, by virtue of their broader practices, have less contact with women seeking home births. Only 24 percent of these respondents have been asked to provide medical backup for home births attended by licensed midwives, and only 18 percent have provided medical care to transferred home birth clients and new-borns as hospital staff or on-call physician. More than one-fifth no longer do obstetrics or have not obtained obstetric privileges at a hospital. Nevertheless, 8 percent have provided medical backup to licensed midwives' clients in the past, and 16 percent would provide such care if asked by a low risk patient in the future. When those who do not do obstetrics are removed from consideration, the proportion of general practitioners willing to provide backup increases to 20 percent.

The survey data support the midwives' belief that physician op-position reflects concern about their qualifications. To help physi-cians evaluate the licensure program, the questionnaire provided information on the requirements for a midwife's license and statistics on prenatal and postpartum transfers by the midwives. The over-whelming majority of obstetricians and general practitioners (88 and 76 percent, respectively) consider the licensure requirements "too lenient." Some of the comments added by respondents contrast the 25 observed and supervised deliveries required for a midwife's li-cense with the 500 to 600 deliveries attended by most obstetricians before certification. Many others question the lack of standardization and the limited duration and nature of midwifery training. For ex-ample, one says that the midwives' "understanding of the mechanics may be acceptable to recognize problems after they occur but they lack the understanding of physiologic functions that would enable them to anticipate problems." Another charges that the "STATIS-TICS [sic] are misleading" and asks: "How many more should have been [transferred]. . . . How do we know how many people (mothers and babies) die not receiving adequate care?"

The midwives' belief that physician opposition to home birth tran-scends the type of attendant also finds support in the survey data. As can be seen in table 7.1, there is substantially more consensus among physician respondents about the risky nature of home birth in partic-ular, and birth in general, than concern that licensed midwives pro-vide inferior maternity care. Respondents' comments on the need to have fetal monitoring and cesarean section equipment on hand reflect their more pathological perspective. One physician writes, for example:

> Catastrophies occur in moments in obstetrics. Maternal and perinatal mortalities have been declining over the past 50 years, all because of increased availability of specialized care centers. By backtracking with home births, how many more women and children will give up their lives so we can relearn an already self-evident lesson.

Some of the physicians even object to the use of the term *low risk* in the questionnaire, claiming that "there is no low risk delivery."

Nearly three-quarters of the obstetricians and more than half of

Table 7.1 Reasons Given by Obstetricians and General Practitioners for Not Providing Medical Backup for Home Births Attended by Licensed Lay Midwives

I would be hesitant to provide medical backup for a licensed lay midwife because:	Obstetricians	General Practitioners
Home birth is too risky, since homes do not have the technology for intervention when problems arise in labor and delivery	97%	76%
A physician can never really say who is a low risk obstetrical patient until after the delivery	97	72
I might be sued after a stillbirth or birth injuries	90	82
My malpractice insurance might not cover me	65	81
It might encourage couples to have their babies at home	72	56
Licensed lay midwives provide inferior maternity care	71	36
I might be ostracized by my peers	34	34
I might risk losing my hospital privileges	24	32

the general practitioners have been asked to deliver home births in the past. In view of their perspective on birth, it is not surprising that only 4 percent of obstetricians and 36 percent of general practitioners have done so. Only 7 percent of obstetricians and one-quarter of the general practitioners would consider such a practice in the future. Physicians so fear the dangers involved in home birth that some add statements such as "Never!!" or "Home deliveries are for pizza" to the standardized answers regarding their willingness to attend home births. One suggests that home birth is as reasonable as "home appendectomies," while another compares it to traveling by horse when cars are available. Forty-four percent of the obstetrician respondents would like the state to prohibit even obstetricians from attending planned home births.

The third reason midwives frequently give when asked why physicians oppose them is that licensed midwives threaten physicians' authority, control, and financial monopoly. Although the questionnaire did not directly address these issues, the survey provides some indirect evidence to support the midwives' claims.

The state's licensure program, described in chapter 5, maintains physicians' authority and control by involving them in the midwifery qualifying examination and as members of the Midwives' Advisory Board. Physicians also participate in the licensure program by providing required laboratory tests, third trimester medical evaluation of clients, and medical backup for labor and delivery. The midwives' guidelines further mandate that midwives urge clients to seek additional prenatal care from a physician and that midwives consult, and be guided by, a physician if any deviations from normal arise. Nevertheless, many physicians comment that licensed midwives do not have enough physician supervision and that physicians have "no control of care or of what happens at a home delivery." Others allude to the issue of control when they note that they support certified nurse-midwives who "work under supervision of obstetricians and in the hospital." In contrast, under Arizona's licensed midwifery program the physician clearly serves as a backup for the client rather than as a supervisor of the midwife. Once a prospective client has passed the medical screening examination, a physician can exercise his or her medical authority only when called upon by a midwife.

Physicians' desire to maintain control also shows in their attitudes

Table 7.2 Percentage of Obstetricians and General Practitioners Who
Support Selected Restrictions on the Practice of Licensed Lay Midwives

Prohibit Licensed Lay Midwives from:	Obstetricians	General Practitioners
Attending nulliparous women	86%	73%
Performing emergency episiotomies	65	56
Suturing first-degree lacerations	61	55
Administering a single dose of an antihemorrhagic before an emergency transfer	49	37

about which procedures midwives should be allowed to perform
(table 7.2). A large majority of both obstetricians and general practitioners would like to stop midwives from attending women having
their first child, and only a minority support the midwives' bid for the
right to perform emergency episiotomies and suture first-degree
tears. Despite physicians' desire to limit the legal scope of midwifery,
however, half the obstetricians and 63 percent of the general practitioners would permit licensed midwives to give an antihemorrhagic
drug before an emergency transfer. Several explain the apparent
contradiction by saying, "If [the midwives] are permitted to deliver
then they should be permitted to do all that is possible in an emergency." The greater support for lifting the restriction on antihemorrhagic drugs also may stem from the qualification that midwives
could administer such drugs only if transferring the client to medical
care.

The midwives believe that physician opposition stems from the
threat that midwives pose to physicians' economic monopoly as well
as the threat to their authority and control. At the time of the survey,
the midwives attended fewer than 2 percent of the births in the state.
The number of home births, however, had been growing rapidly
over the previous seven years. Many of the comments that physicians
add to their questionnaires suggest that it is "foolish to go back to
giving birth like we had to a hundred years ago" when "there is an
adequate number of hospitals and obstetricians within easy reach of

anyone in town" and "adequately trained physicians are in [the] same areas, denied obstetrical privileges." Only 8 percent of obstetricians and 16 percent of general practitioners agree that "to adequately service our population, we need more obstetricians around here." (A few of the obstetricians suggest that there should be fewer general practitioners attending births in their local area as well.) One physician states bluntly, "Economically to allow [midwives] to skim off the easier cases is incorrect. It denies the physician the personal and financial satisfaction to which he is entitled." A retired physician (not included in the statistical analysis) says of his working colleagues, "With the avarice obvious in the profession, they will never 'give'!!" As table 7.3 illustrates, opposition to midwifery is positively correlated with the proportion of a physician's practice that is obstetrical and potentially threatened by home birth midwives.

The findings of the physician survey support the midwives' belief that physician opposition derives from concern about midwives' qualifications, assumptions about the risk of home birth, and the midwives' infringement on medical territory. The survey also reveals another reason for the physicians' reluctance to cooperate—the perceived threat of a malpractice suit. Malpractice suits are the most frequently cited concern of the general practitioners (see table 7.1). Only the closely related concern about the riskiness of birth in general is more salient for obstetricians. The vast majority of both the obstetricians and general practitioners who responded to the questionnaire fear that they might be sued if a complication arose at a

Table 7.3 Physicians' Percentage of Practice That Is Obstetrical by Desire to Prohibit Planned Home Births by Licensed Lay Midwives

Percentage of Practice That Is Obstetrical	Prohibit Planned Home Births by Licensed Midwives
0%	39%
1–24	71
25–49	67
50–74	78
75	83

midwife-attended home birth for which they had agreed to provide medical backup. This fear dominates the physicians' view of midwifery even though the state's program specifically exempts them from a supervisory role over the midwives. The physicians state vehemently that "when a bad result occurs—those with insurance get sued!!" One sums up the prevailing belief: "Obstetrics and Gynecology as a profession is being destroyed by the medical-legal time bomb. Anyone who backs up a lay midwife and exposes himself to the risks that the population represents is a fool."

Concern about the liability involved in providing backup for home births is reinforced by the official statement of the American College of Obstetricians and Gynecologists which explicitly censures home birth:

> Labor and delivery, while a physiologic process, clearly presents potential hazards to both mother and fetus before and during birth. These hazards require standards of safety which are provided in the hospital setting and cannot be matched in the home setting. (1975)

As a result any physician agreeing to attend or provide backup for a home birth is vulnerable to the charge of deviating from good medical practice because he or she is not adhering to official professional standards. According to one legal scholar, a court could find such a doctor negligent because "no physician of standing in the profession would attend a homebirth and therefore, the physician should be absolutely liable for anything that goes on" (Annas, 1976).

Physician concern about malpractice suits extends beyond the issue of home birth. A small number of physicians echo the midwives' charges that hospital obstetrics is characterized by unnecessary, potentially harmful, active interventions but blame malpractice lawyers rather than medical philosophy for this situation. One, for example, says, "I'd be curious to know how many people are aware how much lab tests etc. are ordered to avoid a malpractice suit—I think the public is totally unaware of the effect the lawyers have had." A few respondents even claim sympathy with the home birth midwives and suggest that their own opposition stems solely from the financial burdens imposed by insurance costs. As one physician notes, "I may be more supportive of lay midwives if my malpractice insurance wasn't $23,000."

BIRTH CENTERS: COMPROMISE OR COOPTATION?

Although the vast majority of physicians strongly reject both home birth and lay midwifery, they cannot afford to ignore the widespread consumer dissatisfaction which led to these developments. To reduce the relative attractiveness of home birth for discontented consumers, the American College of Obstetricians and Gynecologists formally endorsed more liberal hospital procedures in 1978 (Interprofessional Task Force on Health Care of Women and Children, 1978). This joint statement by a task force of obstetricians, pediatricians, and nurses called for all hospitals to offer childbirth preparation classes, allow fathers to be present during labor and delivery, loosen restrictions on sibling visits, permit early discharge of mother and baby, and set up "home-like" birth rooms where low risk women can labor, deliver, and recover in one room with family members present. These proposals represent significant changes since most had been widely condemned by physicians as unsafe when first proposed by consumers (Wertz and Wertz, 1977).

Despite previous strong opposition to consumer-proposed changes in obstetrical policies, hospital administrators have been receptive to the task force's suggestions. Hospital birth rooms, in particular, have been promoted as a safe compromise for potential home-birthers (Kerner and Ferris, 1978; Allgaier, 1978; Faxel, 1980; Kieffer, 1980; Dobbs and Shy, 1981).[2] A survey in Washington state just two years after the recommendations found that 63 percent of the hospitals there had opened, or planned to open, a birth room, and that the development of these facilities was positively correlated with the perceived local incidence of home births (Dobbs and Shy, 1981). In California, where the proportion of home births in some suburbs exceeded ten percent in the mid-1970s (*Medical World News*, 1977), the number of alternative birth rooms increased from 3 in 1975 to more than 120 by 1982 (Ostrowski, 1982).

The staff associated with the earliest hospital birth rooms are care-

---

2. Birth rooms also have given hospital administrators a new marketing strategy at a time when competition for consumers has increased greatly. One hospital in Milwaukee which was in danger of closing its obstetrical department due to low usage experienced a seven-fold increase in deliveries after opening a family-centered program (Ruzek, 1980).

ful to point out that "the philosophy of the birthing room is more important than the physical layout" (Faxel, 1980:152). Yet, most hospitals seem to emphasize "interior decorating obstetrics" (Rothman, 1983:4) rather than true philosophical change in developing birth rooms. Hence, home birth advocates view hospital birth rooms as an attempt to coopt dissatisfied consumers by mimicking the physical environment of a home while maintaining medical control, a pathological perspective toward birth, and active medical management (DeVries, 1983; Ruzek, 1980; Rothman, 1981, 1983).

Studies of hospital birth rooms bear out the contention that most offer only the illusion of choice. Contrary to the noninterventionist, wellness perspective of home birth midwives, 92 percent of the birth rooms in Washington hospitals allow narcotics for pain relief, 80 percent allow local anesthesia, and 46 percent allow paracervical blocks. Oxytocin is permitted for labor augmentation in 75 percent of the birth rooms and for initial induction in 46 percent. Seventy-one percent have equipment for electronic fetal monitoring. In fact, the Washington study reveals no differences in labor options available between hospitals with and without birth rooms and few differences in delivery and postpartum options. Hospitals with birth rooms are more likely to allow less controversial options such as the presence of husbands or friends during delivery and not using delivery table stirrups. The more controversial alternative birth options such as husband-assisted delivery, LeBoyer "gentle birth" with bath, gravity or massage in place of newborn suction, and 24-hour rooming-in remain uncommon. Additionally, screened low-risk women who begin their labor in hospital birth rooms are far more likely to be transferred to regular medical care than are women who begin laboring at home. The average transfer rate from birth rooms is 22 percent (DeVries, 1983) compared to the 11 percent reported by Arizona's licensed midwives (chap. 6). In sum, the spread of hospital birth rooms does not seem to reflect any fundamental change in the medical perspective on childbirth. In fact, such major obstetrical interventions as induction, forceps delivery, and cesarean section actually have increased in hospitals at the same time that birth rooms have proliferated.

Along with the development of hospital birth rooms, free-standing birth centers also have emerged to stem interest in home birth (Lubic,

1982). The first was opened in 1975 in New York by the Maternity Center Association in response to increased consumer demand for an alternative to hospital obstetrics. This voluntary health agency previously had established a well-received hospital-based model program in which physicians and certified nurse-midwives cooperated to serve the very poor. The opening of their autonomous Childbearing Center, however, met with considerable physician and hospital opposition. The center aims to provide all consumers maternity care that is "a maxi-home and not a mini-hospital" experience. Birth at the center is managed without "rigid procedures" about labor and delivery positions and without "obstetric modalities and treatments" (Faison et al., 1979:527). The center's emphasis on providing an alternative to standard hospital obstetrics rather than merely extending standard hospital obstetrics to the indigent has led many physicians to view it as an occupational threat rather than as a solution to the perceived risks of planned home births.

Unlike hospital-based birth rooms, free-standing birth centers are officially discouraged by the American College of Obstetricians and Gynecologists and the American Academy of Pediatricians (1983), and physician groups have attempted to deny birth centers access to third-party funding ([Editorial] *American Journal of Nursing,* 1981a, 1981b). Yet, more than 120 free-standing birth centers opened in the last 10 years. Most are run by certified nurse-midwives following the Childbearing Center's philosophy.

While physicians condemn birth centers on the assumption that they present undue medical risks, activists have criticized the centers for coopting consumers seeking changes in childbirth practices by making them part of the "medical establishment from which they are trying to escape" (Eakins, 1984). A collaborative study of 11 selected birth centers reveals less cooptation than found in hospital birth rooms (Bennetts and Lubic, 1982). All centers in this study follow the Maternity Center Association model; care is provided only to the "lowest risk" women, primarily by certified nurse-midwives with physician and hospital backup who are guided by a philosophy of "minimal obstetrical intervention." Only 1 percent of the women at these birth centers are induced compared to the overall rate of 43 percent in hospitals (National Center for Health Statistics, 1984); only 5 percent are delivered with forceps or vacuum extraction compared to 21 percent in hospitals (Haupt, 1982); and only 5 percent end in cesarean sections at a backup hospital compared to the national rate of 20 percent (Taffel et al., 1985). The total transfer rate due to a change in risk status is only 15 percent, which is significantly lower than the average 22 percent rate of in-hospital birth rooms. However, birth centers should not be seen as completely non-medical settings; 40 percent of the labors in the 11 free-standing birth centers are managed with analgesia, anaesthesia, sedatives, hypnotics, or tranquilizers and 38 percent are augmented by artificial rupture of membranes.

The pioneering free-standing birth centers included in this study may well have lower rates of obstetrical intervention than more recently opened centers. The success of the first birth centers and other free-standing, commercial, medical clinics has attracted significant physician interest in spite of their professional associations' opposition. By 1984, physicians were the primary caretakers in 28 percent of the free-standing birth centers (Carey et al., 1984). One boasts: "We lack nothing that a hospital has to deliver a baby except a scalpel for caesareans" (Carey et al., 1984:96). Others run by physicians even offer cesarean sections on the premises.

These developments have led two members of the Maternity Center Association to comment:

> It is paradoxical that, while mainstream obstetrics questions the safety of centres such as those run by the Maternity Center Association, which are scrupulous to offer care only to those at lowest risk, individual practitioners [physicians] are at liberty to develop services which in theory at least entail much greater risk for the families selecting them (Bennetts and Lubic, 1982:11).

Whether the risks are greater remains to be examined, but the services offered in such centers do not reflect the ideology that permeates home birth.

In-hospital birth rooms and free-standing birth centers have the potential to provide a viable compromise for women seeking individualized, holistic, family-centered, maternity care based on a wellness model. Whether they actually do, depends on the philosophical orientation of the care providers. Those that merely transfer the routine, active, medical management of hospital obstetrics to a new location are only another example of the cooptation of childbirth reform attempts, discussed in chapter 2.

Cooptation may well be the fate of all in-hospital and free-standing birth rooms. At the time of this writing, insurance carriers, whose boards of directors are dominated by physicians, have ceased to offer independent certified nurse-midwives and licensed lay midwives separate malpractice insurance premiums based on their risk status. Instead, they are offering insurance only at the rates available to obstetricians, who serve a much higher risk clientele and have a much higher frequency of being sued. The effective unavailability of insurance has forced most free-standing birth centers operated by certified nurse-midwives to close, leaving only those run by physicians.

REFERENCES

Allgaier, A. "Alternative birth centers offer family-centered care. *Hospitals* 52:97, 1978.
American Academy of Pediatrics and American College of Obstetricians and Gynecologists. *Guidelines for Perinatal Care.* Joint Position Statement, 1983.
American College of Obstetricians and Gynecologists. "Statement on home deliveries." *Journal of Nurse-Midwifery* 20:16, 1975.
Annas, George. "Legal aspects of homebirth and other child-birth alternatives," pp. 161–80 in D. Stewart and L. Stewart (eds.), *Safe Alternatives in Childbirth.* Chapel Hill, NC: National Association of Parents and Professionals for Safe Alternatives in Childbirth, 1976.
Bennetts, Anita, and Ruth Watson Lubic. "The free-standing birth centre." *Lancet* 1:11–13, 1982.
Carey, John, Susan Katz, Mary Hager, Barbara Burgower, and Elizabeth Bailey. "The comforts of home: 'Alternative' birthing centers are coming of age." *Newsweek*, November 26:96–99, 1984.
DeVries, Raymond. "Image and reality: An evaluation of Hospital alternative birth centers." *Journal of Nurse-Midwifery* 28:3–9, 1983.
Dobbs, Kathe, and Kirkwood Shy. "Alternative birth rooms and birth options." *Obstetrics and Gynecology* 58:626–30, 1981.
Eakins, Pamela. "The rise of the free standing birth center: Principles and practice." *Women and Health* 9:49–64, 1984.
Editorial. "Midwives tell congressional hearing of widespread opposition by doctors." *American Journal of Nursing* 81:263, 1981a.
Editorial. *American Journal of Nursing* 81:448, 1981b.
Faison, Jere, Bernard Pisani, R. Gordon Douglas, Gene Cranch, and Ruth

Lubic. "The childbearing center: An alternative birth setting." *Obstetrics and Gynecology* 54:527–32, 1979.

Faxel, Ann Marie. "The birthing room concept at Phoenix Memorial Hospital, Part I: Development and eighteen months' statistics." *JOGN Nursing* 9:151–55, 1980.

Haupt, Barbara. "Deliveries in short-stay hospitals: United States, 1980." *Advance Data from Vital and Health Statistics*, No. 83 DHSS Pub. No. (PHS) 82-1250. Hyattsville, MD: Public Health Service, 1982.

Interprofessional Task Force on Health Care of Women and Children. *The Development of Family-Centered Maternity/Newborn Care in Hospitals.* Joint Position Statement, 1978.

Kieffer, Marilyn. "The birthing room concept at Phoenix Memorial Hospital, Part II: Consumer satisfaction during one year," *JOGN Nursing* 9:155–59, 1980.

Kerner, J., and C. B. Ferris. "An alternative birth center in a community teaching hospital." *Obstetrics and Gynecology* 51:371, 1978.

Lubic, Ruth. "The rise of the birth center alternative." *The Nation's Health,* January 7, 1982.

Medical World News. "California: Furor over home births." April 4, 1977.

National Center for Health Statistics. "Trends in maternal and infant health factors associated with low birth weight, United States, 1972 and 1980." *Public Health Reports* 99:162–72, 1984.

Obstetrics and Gynecology News. "ACOG official: Home delivery maternal trauma, child abuse." October 1:1, 1977.

Ostrowski, L. L. *Alternative Birth Centers.* Berkeley, CA: Department of Health Services, 1982.

Rothman, Barbara. "Awake and aware, or false consciousness: The cooptation of childbirth reform in America, pp. 150–80 in Shelly Romalis (ed.), *Childbirth Alternatives to Medical Control.* Austin: University of Texas Press, 1981.

Rothman, Barbara. "Anatomy of a compromise: Nurse-midwifery and the rise of the birth center." *Journal of Nurse Midwifery* 28:3–7, 1983.

Ruzek, Sheryl. "Medical response to women's health activities: Conflict, accommodation and cooptation." *Researching the Sociology of Health Care* 1:335–54, 1980.

Taffel, Selma, Paul Placek, and Mary Moien. "One Fifth of 1983 U.S. Births by Cesarean Section." *American Journal of Public Health* 75:190, 1985.

Wertz, Richard, and Dorothy Wertz. *Lying-In: A History of Childbirth in America.* New York: Free Press, 1977.

CHAPTER 8

THE MIDWIVES' RESPONSE
TO RESTRICTIONS
AND OPPOSITION

As chapter 7 shows, physicians are vociferously and almost uniformly opposed to home birth midwifery. Yet midwives need physicians' cooperation to practice safely. In the absence of such cooperation, most midwives find it difficult to arrange essential medical backup for the occasional unexpected complications that develop in spite of client screening. At the same time, opposition from physicians has kept most lay midwives from gaining legal recognition and has forced them to work under the threat of prosecution. In states where legal recognition has been obtained, midwives have exchanged the vulnerability of illegality for restrictive licensure under medical control, as discussed in chapter 5. Moreover, midwives' exposure to physicians' strong disapproval presents a continual challenge to the midwives' image of themselves as competent professionals providing a valuable service. This chapter explores how midwives deal with these legal, practical, and psychological dilemmas caused by physician opposition.

WORKING OUTSIDE THE LAW

Most lay midwives work in a legal limbo—neither clearly prohibited nor regulated by current state statutes. In such circumstances the legality of their practice is subject to the vagaries of law enforcement officials' interpretations of the scope of medical practice and responsibility for perinatal mortality. These midwives work with the recognition that they could be charged with practicing medicine without a license or worse:

> If anything goes wrong at a home birth you are in fear of being prosecuted. You could be charged with murder. And deaths do happen. It is part of birth. . . . It doesn't matter how ideal birthing services are, no matter where it is, you will get some deaths.

Few are ever prosecuted for attending home births, but these fears are not unfounded. A cease and desist order issued during the interview period to one midwife in the northeastern state reminded others in her area of their legal vulnerability.

Unlicensed midwives who are registered nurses express additional concern that they might jeopardize that credential. Most who work in hospitals do not tell their supervisors or co-workers that they attend home births. They avoid interacting as midwives with the hospitals where they work and fear discovery in an emergency transfer.

The unlicensed midwives' self-described "paranoia" extends beyond a concern for their own vulnerability to fear of the potential repercussions on their families. One, for example, has moved all belongings out of her house several times following hospital transfers when she feared that possible prosecution would jeopardize her family's limited assets. Another described her terror when going to the hospital with a depressed baby:

> I was resuscitating the baby the whole way to the hospital. While this was going on, part of me said, "Oh my God. . . ." I realized that [if the outcome was bad] that would be not only heavy for me but for my family. Maybe I could live with it, but, if it became this big case? The baby ended up being fine and everything else, but in some ways I said "Hey. . . ."

Several of the more affluent midwives mention that their husbands, although philosophically supportive of their practice, worry about their financial as well as legal liability. One of them worked with physicians to "mollify" her husband. Now that these physicians no longer attend home births, her husband wants her to quit unless she can obtain malpractice insurance. As a compromise, she limits herself to attending the births of friends and previous clients.

The absence of clear regulatory guidelines makes unlicensed midwives particularly vulnerable to prosecution and conviction by the media. A popular magazine, for example, ran an article about a Massachusetts midwife titled, "Friendly Acquaintances: The relationship was a success. The baby was stillborn" (Kahn, 1982). The article acknowledged that the unlicensed midwife was not working as a midwife in the case; that she had only seen the couple once before when they asked her to serve as a labor coach/patient advocate for their planned hospital birth; and that she only came to the house in the middle of the night as moral support after the woman, suffering cramplike pains several weeks before her due date, called her obstetrician and was told that she probably had a virus and should visit the office the next morning. Nevertheless, the article insinuated that the midwife was responsible for the stillbirth by noting that the midwife suggested the woman soak in a tub to relieve her cramps while the midwife rested and that the woman gave birth precipitously an hour and a half later.

Unlicensed midwives cope with their legal vulnerability in a variety of ways. All stress the limitations of their services to prospective clients. All try to prevent problems and to deal with problems such as tears and hemorrhages without involving medical personnel. Some have clients sign informed choice statements releasing the midwife of legal responsibility, while a few limit their practice to friends. At least one uses an alias for her midwifery practice. Some claim to be only friends when accompanying a transferred client to a hospital, while a few report accompanying their clients to the hospital door but not inside.

At the other extreme are the majority of unlicensed midwives, who practice openly, insist that their clients tell their prenatal physicians that they plan a midwife-attended home birth, and assertively acknowledge their role to physicians. Some have an account with a laboratory for prenatal screening. These midwives believe:

> If you act as if there is something shady going on, they are going to assume it. But, if I go right in as though I am legitimate and I am to be accepted as an equal with you, or as a partner in this birth team, they accept that.

One midwife's experience illustrates the positive effect of a confident attitude in dealing with hospital staff considered hostile to home birth:

There was an obstetrician whose nurse had a home birth. He gave her a lot of negative—how could she do this? I had a woman who was not in labor but she was at home and the cord came out. . . . I instructed her as to what to do. Of course, the ambulance took her to the closest hospital. . . . I appeared there right away . . . with all my records, very official, you know. [The obstetrician who was performing the emergency cesarean] said, "Oh, tell the midwife I'll be right out." I thought, "Oh, this is it; they are going to arrest me." He came out and said, "Well, we got the baby out in only 17 minutes." And, I realized that he was trying to say that I'd done a good job with this. I started working with him more as a colleague. He said, "I know you're the one that delivered my nurse's baby." It was all right then. Even the pediatrician came out a couple of times to tell me of the progress . . . and this was the hospital that everyone was afraid of!

To gain support for their work, half the interviewed unlicensed midwives have joined the Midwives Alliance of North America, a new voluntary association of certified nurse- and lay midwives. Many have spoken at health fairs and to school, childbirth, and other community groups. Some have given interviews to newspaper, radio, and television reporters. Several have served on consumer advisory committees for their local hospitals, while some have met with paramedic groups. One serves on a committee convened by a local district attorney to discuss establishing a program to credential lay midwives.

Perhaps the most important response of these unlicensed midwives to their vulnerable position has been the development of the voluntary credential program described in chapter 5. The development of this program has accompanied efforts to establish midwifery licensure, even though many of the midwives wonder whether they could accept the inevitable restrictions on their practice that licensure would entail. It is the prospect of legal protection, however, along with the belief that licensure will improve interactions with the medical community, that make licensure attractive to the majority in spite of restrictions.

NEGOTIATING THE LICENSURE SYSTEM

Licensure frees midwives from the fear of prosecution for practicing medicine or nurse-midwifery without a license. In exchange for this protection, midwives must limit their practices to abide by their legal restrictions, as discussed in chapter 5.

The midwives accept these restrictions as long as they feel that their clients' health is not threatened. The restrictive nature of Arizona's licensure, however, creates a dilemma for state midwives. In emergencies, Arizona midwives have performed episiotomies, and those who have documented the need for so doing have not been disciplined. Some illegally carry antihemorrhagic drugs. Others suggest that their clients obtain an antihemorrhagic prescription for self-administration in an emergency. A more frequent problem is perineal lacerations, which Arizona midwives cannot suture. If the tear is small and likely to heal with proper care, the midwives often have the client decide whether she wants to be transferred to a physician for sutures. Unless necessary, the midwives want to avoid the expense, the physical discomfort, and the psychological trauma of disturbing the family bonding and exposing the woman to potentially hostile medical staff.

The midwives have lobbied their state Advisory Committee for several years for the legal right to do emergency episiotomies, to administer a single dose of an antihemorrhagic drug in an emergency, and to suture minor lacerations and emergency episiotomies. At the time of the interviews, most midwives were optimistic that the Department of Health Services would soon change their guidelines. In the three years since then, no changes have been made despite the hiring of new directors of maternity services increasingly sympathetic to the midwives' requests. Changing the guidelines would necessitate an open discussion in the legislature, where state health officials fear that several members committed to deregulation might be able to scuttle the licensure system. As described in chapter 4, one of these legislators did succeed in temporarily loosening the training requirements. As a result, revision has been postponed.

The licensed midwives' association has lobbied against deregulation and in favor of retaining a strict licensure law. Only one midwife, whose license had been suspended, supports deregulation. The midwives' association fears that deregulation would lower the standard of midwifery care and consequently fuel physician opposition to midwifery. One midwife states, for example: "I just think it is ridiculous to have people who are not trained and who've not been tested that they can at least perform at a minimal level of competence be allowed to deliver babies. Because there are lives involved." Another licensed midwife explains that deregulation is "a very bad thing because I feel it will put us right back to where we were before we started to become a little more accepted and trusted by the medical profession." Although the licensed midwives generally sympathize with the concerns of unlicensed midwives and recognize their common origins, they cannot afford to align themselves too closely with them. Instead, as the next section discusses, they must focus on gaining the support of physicians.

DEALING WITH PHYSICIANS

The problems posed by physician opposition and the responses to them among licensed and unlicensed midwives are more alike than different. Contrary to the unlicensed midwives' expectations, the major problem faced by the licensed midwives is not the restrictions on their practice, but the general unwillingness of physicians to provide needed prenatal screening and medical backup. Although a few licensed and unlicensed midwives have long-standing arrangements with physicians who provide prenatal screening and medical backup, most must continually search for a sympathetic physician. As one states: "I try to have contact with the physicians and establish a personal rapport with them. It sometimes works. It sometimes doesn't. And sometimes, it seems that we've had a rapport established and then all of a sudden I hear that they are going to have the next midwife that they see arrested."

Many midwives can obtain backup support only from marginal practitioners—osteopaths, semiretired physicians, and physicians who lack hospital privileges. For example: "The only doctor who would work with us . . . doesn't have hospital privileges. He's a kind of retired obstetrician . . . [and] a Seventh Day Adventist. . . . He doesn't prescribe any medications. He just works with herbs and stuff. [Since he doesn't have hospital privileges], if we ran into a complication we had to go to the emergency room and take whoever was there."

Midwives who cannot find any sympathetic physicians or whose backups lack hospital privileges must rely on public hospitals for any needed medical care. One midwife describes the resulting problems: "We are not able to turn our patients over to optimum obstetricians.

We have to turn them over to residents. And most often these residents are not of the best quality, and that is a real heartbreak—the way you see some of these babies being delivered, you could almost have done better at home." All midwives try to avoid hospitals with the most hostile staff. One explains how "we're really careful what hospital we take the ladies into because some of them just have such negative attitudes. It's like you are throwing a poor lady into a lion's den.

Midwives faced with this dilemma sometimes put off transferring a client to medical care until the need to do so is inescapable. In other situations, midwives transfer clients before it is clear that such care is needed, to avoid angering a backup physician if the problem becomes more serious. One midwife declares, "The more I practice, the more I practice defensively." Another states, "You get a much better relationship with the medical profession if you are overly cautious.

The problems of obtaining and keeping medical backup also affect the criteria that midwives use to screen potential clients. The midwives have learned that physicians frequently regard transfers as evidence against home birth rather than as evidence that midwives recognize incipient problems and obtain timely medical assistance. As a result midwives are hesitant to accept marginal cases even if they fall within established low risk norms or, in Arizona, within the state's regulatory guidelines. Such cases are less problematic for those licensed midwives whose clients have an individual physician serving as backup, since the midwives can call them for advice and, sometimes, continue care at home under the physician's authority in circumstances where other clients relying on public hospital staff would have to be transferred.

Several midwives explain that their screening criteria vary depending upon the level of hostility among local physicians in the various areas they serve. To try to ensure that interactions with physicians proceed smoothly, the midwives try to screen out clients who seem hostile toward or afraid of physicians or hospitals. All counsel their clients on the need to act cooperatively if they must be transferred to medical care.

To improve their legal status and their access to backup medical care, the midwives try to encourage good relations with physicians. They feel they "have responsibility to make sure this movement looks

legitimate." A few unlicensed midwives note that the "political climate" is the only reason they refuse women who previously have had
cesarean sections. One insists on using cord clamps because "a cord
clamp looks better to a doctor [than a] dirty shoelace." Many attempt
to foster an interpersonal style which will placate physicians and encourage their support. The midwives—generally rather strong and
independent women—try to act in a compliant and nonthreatening
fashion in their interaction with physicians. They recognize that "if
you give them a hard time [at the hospital], they'll throw you out" and
clients' care might suffer. Most feel it is wiser to "fade into the wall-
paper." As one midwife explains, "The relationship with the doctor
means a lot to you. . . . You [have] got to really be nice to them if
you're going to get anything you want because they're not going to do
it if you show anger." The midwives try to avoid calling physicians for
advice at inconvenient hours. Most will not question a physician's
judgment unless they feel their client is seriously endangered. Even
in those circumstances they try to do so tactfully and out of the client's
hearing. As a result, some report silently watching inept care leading
to unnecessary blood loss, lacerations, or depressed babies.

One midwife who has adopted a very professional, conservative
style reports using a wide variety of tactics to develop good relations
with physicians:

> I send flowers to the labor and to delivery nurses, thanking them for the
> effort put forth. . . . I write letters of thanks for the nice hospitality
> shown. . . . I've written letters [to physicians] explaining the home birthing
> movement and credentializing it. I make personal visits to doctors intro-
> ducing them to what's going on and encouraging them to be very careful
> about who they will see for home birthing. I have written letters to hospital
> administrators. . . . I do [so] much P.R. . . . because I like the medical field
> to see that this is the type of midwife that they don't have to be fearing. This
> is the type of responsible person that is not going to compromise them.

Some midwives send their backup physicians copies of their records
after each delivery to stress that they are part of the health care
"team" rather than competitors. One admits that she keeps "quite
thick records . . . to integrate myself with the medical establishment
more than anything else." Many now keep their case records on
forms similar to those used in local hospitals. These midwives have
learned that, in the event of a transfer to medical care, hospital staff

respect their knowledge about their clients more when it is presented in a familiar way.

As the midwives gain experience, they learn that their personal appearance, as well as their style of interaction, can affect physicians' attitudes toward them. As a result, several report modifying their style of dress to gain the respect of physicians and hospital staff: "I was from the hippie era. And I didn't dress so nice and a lot of people were offended by that when I was a student midwife. . . . So I've started changing that since I've been licensed." Another explains: "If I think I'm going to go to the hospital . . . , I put on some white pants. If I think it's goint to be a transport, I dress a lot straighter."

In sum, physician opposition pressures midwives to practice and to present themselves in a more conservative style. Many of those who do not do so find themselves overtly or covertly accused of hindering the acceptance of midwifery. For example, one midwife states: "I think the way some of [the midwives] present themselves, myself included, is not always good for licensed midwifery. Some of our midwives [have] got 58 layers of big plumpy skirts and haggy looking blouses and no bras and high top tennis shoes. It doesn't do anything to instill confidence from regular medical people in what we're doing." Conversely, those who adopt the most conservative styles may be suspected of selling out. These tensions arise because the midwives realize their fates are tied. Yet these same tensions make it more difficult for the midwives to join together in common cause. Despite their attempts to placate physicians, all the midwives know that the vast majority of physicians oppose midwife-attended home births.

MAINTAINING SELF-IMAGE AND PHILOSOPHY

The need for medical backup means that all midwives must occasionally interact with physicians. All midwives have some plan for transfer to medical care if complications develop. Most require that their clients make arrangements with a physician. The licensed midwives legally are required to accompany their clients if medical aid is needed, and almost all the unlicensed midwives also do so. As one unlicensed midwife says, "We go in with the people and take all of the grief and everything . . . we are no longer responsible technically but it's our own private responsibility to them."

These interactions with physicians ensure that all midwives are well aware of medical views regarding home birth and midwifery. Those who have found one or two sympathetic physicians will often restrict their clients to these backups to reduce exposure to negative attitudes. For the rest, the continual process of searching for physicians willing to provide backup exposes midwives to the disdain of physicians. Even among physicians willing to provide backup, the cooperation is usually reluctant: "They do this 'spiel' about 'we're not responsible for what happens to you and we don't really support homebirth, but if that is what you're going to do, that is what you're going to do, and you understand that we are not going to attend your birth at home.'" Moreover, even those with sympathetic backup physicians may come into contact with other, more hostile, medical personnel if a transfer to a hospital is required.

Almost every midwife reports at least one incident where a physician charged her or her client with foolishness for attempting a home birth. These incidents are emotionally traumatic for the midwife as well as the mother. One describes how one physician in her area who provides backup

> sometimes just went off the wall and scared the hell out of the ladies, telling them that they were taking the babies' life into their own hands and were at great risk and that the midwives practicing in this area were incompetent. So, we would get a lady who is eight months pregnant, who we would be doing prenatal care for, who had really built up a relationship of love and trust in us, who is now scared to death. . . . Some people he doesn't hassle . . . but he has really, really done a job on some of our ladies which I think is a misuse of his power.

Another midwife describes the experience of a woman whom she transferred to have a minor tear stitched: "She was fine; the baby was fine; but while the physician was stitching, he kept telling her about the risks she had taken." Other midwives claim that hospital personnel have told recuperating home birth mothers that "home birth is akin to walking across the street blindfolded" and "you did the stupidest thing you ever could have done in your life and you might have killed your baby and died yourself."

More serious, although rare, are midwives' reports of incidents in which physicians punish mothers for having home births by refusing assistance or inflicting unnecessary pain on them during examination and treatment. For example, one midwife says that she had to have an out-of-area doctor call her local hospital to insist that they treat a woman transferred there in an emergency with a declining fetal heart rate early in labor. Another claims that a physician insisted on a spinal anesthetic to repair a second-degree tear and during the procedure, "he was saying 'now if you had been a good girl and hadn't had your baby at home, we wouldn't be having to do this and you wouldn't have gotten me out of bed' and it was really . . . flat out punishment."

Once a midwife transfers her client to a hospital, the midwife must make the transition from being in charge to being clearly subordinate. If permitted, she may function as a consumer advocate. She has, however, no official role and little power to maintain nonmedical definitions of childbirth or to minimize active medical management. In this setting the midwives must acknowledge and accept physicians' authority and the prevailing medical model of childbirth.

Recognition of physicians' extreme disapproval presents a serious challenge to midwives' view of themselves and their work. As one reports: "I'd have to say it [physician disapproval] affects me. I guess when you have someone who is questioning what you do, you question yourself. And so it's undermining. It doesn't do anything for my confidence and it does undermine my confidence." Another, who is phasing out her midwifery practice, describes how doctors "make me feel like I'm an inch tall sometimes. . . . It makes me not want to do births that much." Two others who have reduced drastically their unlicensed practice say that physicians' negative attitudes during transfers and consults make it harder for them to "bring [up] all the information that I had . . . because I was anxious." Even among the licensed midwives, these same pressures led 9 of the 27 to begin training in nursing or nurse-midwifery by early 1987. Although they still believe in the value of their work as midwives, they have tired of the strain of being marginal, though legal, practitioners and want to increase their status and the legal scope of their practice.

Challenges to midwives' beliefs are particularly threatening if they come when a planned home birth has failed. Sooner or later, all midwives encounter a mother who fails to progress, tears, or hemorrhages; a physically depressed or traumatized baby; or a stillbirth. As discussed in chapter 6, such incidents occur less frequently in carefully screened home births than hospital births, but they do happen.

The midwives recognize the potential for difficulties to arise in childbirth and always explain to clients that a small percentage of their cases require medical aid. But they emphasize that the hazards of typical hospital obstetric care outweigh the dangers of a properly screened and managed home birth.

Despite this intellectual awareness of potential difficulties, midwives and parents still face disappointment whenever a planned home birth develops problems. The need to transfer a client demonstrates that the midwife is unable, despite careful screening, to predict whether a woman can safely deliver at home. In these circumstances, the midwife reviews her actions and the woman's history searching for explanations. If, simultaneously, medical staff castigate the midwife for what they consider her stupidity in not recognizing the inherent and unpredictable dangers of childbirth, the midwife may experience a crisis of confidence in her ability and philosophy. This situation can, and sometimes does, pressure midwives to adopt a more medicalized view of childbirth and more conservative practices.

The impact of physicians' attitudes on midwives' beliefs is considerably more limited than this discussion might suggest, however, since the midwives discount physicians' views in several ways. First, midwives note the self-serving nature of physician opposition. The midwives recognize that they financially threaten obstetricians because medical care costs approximately four times the price of midwifery care. One midwife claims that her husband "figured out how much money I cost the local obstetricians and hospital and it was one-quarter of a million dollars."

Although the proportion of home births is minuscule, the number has increased steadily. Concurrently, obstetricians' income has been squeezed by the oversupply of physicians coupled with exorbitant malpractice insurance costs. In one city, where physician opposition is strongest and most widespread, several of the midwives voice similar opinions: "There are too many OBs in [this area and we] . . . would definitely take away a certain population, especially if the population felt that doctors were giving approval and giving good back-up."

The midwives suggest that physicians also may disparage midwives in order to bolster their own self-image:

> So much of this is all ego, you know. Their egos are real insulted that here's this crop of people coming along and saying, "we've never gone to school, we're self-educated, but we can do just as good as you." And here's [*sic*] all these consumers that are going "yeah, we'll go to you [the midwife] and not to you [the physicians]." There's a lot of ego in this whole thing, and then they have to . . . make up things in their mind to justify [their opposition to midwifery].

Another midwife notes: "When doctors get right down to it, when they are honest enough, then they would really have to answer we [midwives] are not a threat [to them]. It's the fact that the pregnant consumer is not satisfied with what they are doing, and we are simply providing a viable alternative."

The midwives also discount physician opposition by noting that physicians hold distorted information about midwifery: "They stereotype us. . . . [They think] that we don't know anything . . . , that we are willing to handle things that we are not willing to handle— breeches, hemorrhages—that we don't know our limitations." Licensed midwives additionally stress that no matter what gaps existed in their initial training, they all have proved their knowledge and skills through a qualifying examination. Yet, physicians continue to regard them as untrained: "[I] go into the hospital and I introduce myself. I say, 'I'm a licensed midwife,' and I hear that person I just said that to turn around [and say] 'the *lay* midwife is with her.'" They view physicians' continued use of the term *lay midwife* as an insult and as a reflection of physicians' misinformation about licensed midwifery.

Both the licensed and unlicensed midwives suggest that physicians' notions about childbirth are distorted by their skewed experiences. Since physicians serve as a much higher risk group than do midwives, they tend, in the midwives' opinion, to overestimate the dangers of childbirth. Similarly, the midwives believe that physicians overestimate the dangers of home birth because they see home birth mothers and babies only when difficulties arise.

The midwives maintain their self-esteem in the face of physician opposition not only by discounting physicians' motives and knowledge but also by focusing on the benefits of home birth, the need to maintain this alternative to medical care, and the purity of their own motives. As described in chapter 3, the midwives believe that hospital births present greater physical and psychological risks than do home births. The midwives point to the high rates of cesarean sections, episiotomies, inductions, and drug use as examples of unnecessary and harmful medical interventions. The midwives' primary aim is to provide a low intervention, family-centered alternative for normal childbirth. They assert that by relying upon the natural birth process and natural forms of assistance, they not only provide a safer alternative in the normal situation but also strengthen family bonds and give mothers a sense of strength and accomplishment.

The midwives' commitment to providing this service is strong enough that they will take personal risks to do so. Most of the unlicensed midwives regard their practice as illegal because of its treatment in state courts. Several describe their midwifery work as a kind of civil disobedience. These midwives believe that "there are higher laws than the ones that people make" and that "every woman should have the right to choose who they want to have with them when they give birth [and] wherever they want to give birth within reason." Only two of the unlicensed midwives would cease practicing in the state if faced with explicit legislative or judicial prohibition. Six others would think about stopping depending on the nature of the law and whether they had young children. Among Arizona's licensed midwives, 62 percent say that they would continue to practice if midwifery were made illegal.

While the midwives discount physicians' objections as self-serving, they can provide strong evidence that their own motives are pure, which further bolsters their self-esteem and belief system. One of the unlicensed midwives asserts: "We're risking everything. Every delivery I do . . . , I'm risking my home which is all I have. So it really puts you on the line. Obviously, it's not the money." Another says, "There's no money in it. . . . I feel like I'm really doing a service for somebody." A former nun comments that midwifery is more a "vocation" than a profession. Midwifery has only recently become financially profitable for any of the midwives. Only 4 of the 50 reported a yearly income from midwifery above $10,000, while most continue to

obtain only a marginal income from their time-consuming and physically demanding work. This lack of financial motive is reflected in
the midwives' disapproval of and occasional refusal to accept clients
who want a home birth simply to save money.

Midwives' ability to retain their beliefs is made easier by their large
network of supporters, including friends, clients, other midwives,
and national organizations. Since the midwives generally interact
only with others who share their values, their perceptions of general
social attitudes are colored. Although the midwives occasionally hear
that clients' friends and families fear the dangers of home birth, they
rarely have to deal with these individuals directly. Only five of the
licensed midwives and seven of the unlicensed report that their own
parents did not approve of their midwifery practice, and some of
these have limited contact with their parents because of previous
nontraditional life choices.

Within their social networks, midwives are seen as performing a
needed and highly valued service. Every midwife reports that all or
almost all of her friends supported her decision to enter midwifery.
When, for example, one midwife faced legal harassment instigated
by local physicians, her neighbors organized an arts fair to raise money for her legal costs. In fact, the midwives report they sometimes
have trouble developing normal social relationships because others
romanticize their work and admire them excessively. Many expressed sentiments similar to the midwife who complained, "People
want to put you on a pedestal as the 'Great Earth Mother.' God forbid
you should light up a cigarette."

Thus, although physician hostility forces midwives to evaluate and
confront the potential hazards of home birth, they can focus on its
benefits and on their record of successes. As chapter 6 has shown, the
statistics on maternal and perinatal mortality demonstrate that licensed midwives, at least, provide an excellent standard of care. The
midwives are aware and proud of these statistics. The women also
stress that midwife-assisted home birth remains the most common
mode of maternity care throughout the world. As one notes, "Our
country is so unrepresentative of the world. . . . Ninety-five percent
of the people alive in the world today were born at home." The
midwives are well aware that countries exist which rely on midwife-

attended hospital birth and have far better morbidity and mortality outcomes than the United States.

TEMPTATION, LEGITIMATION, AND COOPTATION

Midwives, like other alternative practitioners, have strong motivations for seeking legitimation. Yet legitimation presents dangers. Most crucially, how does one obtain legitimation without sacrificing the principles which led to the search for an alternative in the first place?

In order to have their views accepted, persons promoting new ideas must first develop some credibility and respectability among those currently in power. To do so, innovators must downplay the difference between their views and practices and normative views and practices. As described in this chapter, both licensed and unlicensed midwives have adopted a more conservative practice style and self-presentation in an attempt to develop greater support among physicians. An alternative strategy is to suggest that these new ideas and practices logically derive from more generally accepted principles. Midwives have appealed with some success to state legislatures on the basis of the American belief in the right to privacy and freedom of choice.

In the short run, at least, innovative ideas rarely are adopted intact by mainstream society. As a result, marginal acceptance means that persons promoting new alternatives constantly face psychological and intellectual challenges to their belief system. Physician hostility not only has hampered midwives' ability to provide a true alternative but also has forced them to question the quality of the care they do provide. Although most midwives continue to believe in themselves and their work, some have begun questioning seriously their ability and philosophy; probably none is unaffected by the pressure to adopt a view of childbirth which highlights the potential for problems.

The dilemma posed by the need to obtain physician cooperation while avoiding cooptation is one faced by all alternative practitioners from osteopaths (New, 1960) and pharmacists (Cain and Kahn, 1971) to chiropractors (Rosenthal, 1981) and chiropodists (Larkin, 1983). As long as physicians retain their current level of professional and social dominance, any change in health care delivery will come on their terms.

REFERENCES

Cain, Rosalyn, and Joel Kahn. "The pharmacist as a member of the health team." *American Journal of Public Health* 11:2220–28, 1971.

Kahn, E. J. "Friendly acquaintances: The relationship was a success. The baby was stillborn." *Boston Magazine,* September:164–66, 1982.

Larkin, Gerald. *Occupational Monopoly and Modern Medicine.* New York: Tavistock, 1983.

New, Peter Kong-ming. "The osteopathic student: A study in dilemma," pp. 413–21 in E. Gartly Jaco (ed.), *Patients, Physicians and Illness.* New York: Free Press, 1958.

Rosenthal, Saul. "Marginal or mainstream: Two studies of contemporary chiropractors." *Sociological Focus* 14:271–85, 1981.

CHAPTER 9
THE BIRTH AND DEATH
OF INDEPENDENT MIDWIFERY:
BRITAIN, AUSTRALIA,
AND NEW ZEALAND

In chapter 1 we argue that the decline of midwifery in the United States is the unique result of the interaction between the medicalization of childbirth and the delayed regulation of health care occupations within a heterogeneous, decentralized, democratic culture. In no other society except Canada[1] has this ancient female occupation been virtually eliminated as it was by the mid-twentieth century in the United States. Yet the seeds of change were planted in the English motherland before the American colonies won their independence.

Unlike on the European continent, no municipal regulation or training programs were established for British midwives in the seventeenth or eighteenth century.[2] Until the turn of the twentieth century, British midwives remained unorganized and unregulated except for the moral control of episcopal licensing. They were fully responsible for normal births and were required to call a barber-

---

1. Although lay midwives practice throughout Canada, physicians are the only individuals who may attend births legally, with the exception of nurses working in remote rural areas without medical assistance (Hinds, 1985:46). Two provinces (Ontario and Quebec) are currently considering proposals for the introduction of legal midwifery.

2. The following discussion of British midwifery draws heavily on Donnison's (1977) excellent, detailed history.

surgeon to intervene with his instruments only in abnormal cases. Training during this period consisted primarily of apprenticeship, although male midwives and physicians associated with the new lying-in hospitals provided some lectures for midwives in the eighteenth century.

Men who specialized in midwifery first appeared in Britain in the early seventeenth century. This incursion into what had been an all-female field was helped along when Peter Chamberlen, a male midwife, modified the levers used by barber-surgeons into forceps. This new instrument sometimes gave the Chamberlen family an alternative to sacrificing either the mother or infant, as usually happened in abnormal cases. Its dissemination in the eighteenth century among other male midwives provided a technological basis for an eventual alliance with surgeons. The rigid British guild system and prevailing gender norms prevented female midwives from having access to forceps or other instruments and, consequently, excluded them from the fraternity of physicians.

By 1750 Forbes (1971:354) estimates that there were hundreds of male midwives in London. With the help of philanthropists, some established lying-in hospitals for the poor to gain the clinical experience necessary to support their expanded claim to normal, as well as abnormal, childbirth among the affluent. Their clientele was growing at the time of the American Revolution.

Socially elite British and European physicians opposed male midwifery as beneath the dignity of professional men (Donnison, 1977:47). Even the less elite surgeons accepted only reluctantly their evolving alliance with male midwives. Such opposition to attending childbirth did not exist among most Colonial American physicians, few of whom could claim professional status based on family lineage or afford to give up the potential income of midwifery (Starr, 1982:39, 85). Neither did it exist in Britain's other English-speaking colonies of Australia and New Zealand. Physicians in these two countries, as in the United States, had greater vested interests in eliminating midwives than did physicians in Britain.

This chapter compares and contrasts the evolution of midwifery in Britain, Australia, and New Zealand with that of the United States. The histories show that the current status of midwives in each country is a product not only of physician status and interests but also of economic development, social stratification, government structure, the timing of regulation, the degree of integration with British medicine, and geographic barriers to health care delivery. In spite of these historical differences, the data suggest a convergence in the role of midwives in these countries.

GREAT BRITAIN

The Rise of Obstetrics

British physicians' opposition to attending childbirth began to erode in the first half of the nineteenth century. During this period the traditional physician/surgeon/apothecary hierarchy of English medicine that placed professions over crafts and crafts over trades was changing into a two-tiered system of elite consultants (specialists) and general practitioners. Starr (1982:78) attributes this structural change to the expansion of a middle-class market for medical care as in the United States, the upgrading of apothecary education, and the infusion of French medical advances such as pelvimetry which compelled even elite physicians to perform manual procedures previously delegated to surgeons.

Arney (1982:24) additionally argues that the transfer of French technology to monitor pregnancy, without the French ideology of the inherent normalcy of childbirth, propelled British medical practitioners to usurp from midwives the power to define normal and abnormal. When combined with forceps, monitoring technology provided physicians with techniques which, when used judiciously, could improve the outcomes of abnormal cases. This development gradually made the new field of obstetrics more palatable to physicians. Attendance at childbirth became actively pursued by emerging middle-class general practitioners who, like American physicians earlier, needed to build a practice in a highly competitive market. Their clientele grew at the expense of midwives who were increasingly limited to serving the poor.

The growing legitimacy of obstetrics as a medical field was evident in the Medical Act of 1858. In that year, the newly formed General Council for Medical Education published the first Medical Register of practitioners holding diplomas from recognized institutions. Concurrently, the Royal Colleges established optional examinations for men in midwifery. Donnison (1977:42–56) asserts that the optional nature of the midwifery examinations until 1886 and the ban against electing practicing male midwives to the Fellowship of the Colleges of Physicians and Surgeons indicate the continuing low status of obstetrics at this time. Nevertheless, the optional examinations represented the first step toward eventual respectability and formal acceptance of male childbirth attendants. Attempts by the small, newly formed Obstetrical Association of Midwives and the short-lived Female Medical Society to have female midwives listed in the Medical Register did not succeed for another half century.

The Battle to Subordinate Midwives

By the turn of the twentieth century, the battle for the right to organize, register, and regulate British midwives had spanned several hundred years. Male midwives first petitioned the king and Privy Council in the seventeenth century for control over their female peers. Their efforts proved unsuccessful since childbirth at that time was still considered a nonmedical event best left to women judged to be of good character by the Church.

As the power of the Church waned during the eighteenth century the traditional system of episcopal licensing lost authority. Perhaps more important for the future of midwifery, midwives in subsequent decades were increasingly drawn from the lower class; Victorian norms dictated that genteel women should not work, especially at something so indelicate as midwifery. The unprotected, unorganized, often illiterate, lower-class midwives of the early and middle nineteenth century were powerless to ward off the forces pushing for medicalization of childbirth. Perceiving an opportunity to increase their domain, the apothecaries, the new Obstetrical Society (a group of male childbirth attendants), and the British Nurses' Association each lobbied for authority over midwives. All proposed to improve standards of midwifery. Their repeated attempts were blocked by a diverse group of opponents: elite physicians who still considered childbirth to be undignified women's work, feminists who viewed the proposed restrictions on practice as subordination, members of Parliament who felt that subordinating midwives would violate the principle of free trade, and general practitioners who wanted to exclude rather than supervise midwives.

Despite both the failure to subordinate or exclude British midwives and the traditional opposition to male attendants, men increasingly gained control over childbirth. Their eventual domination reflected the effects of class consciousness and normative gender roles. As in the United States, middle-class males took over the majority of births in affluent areas by the second half of the nineteenth century. They were aided by the stereotype of midwives as lower-class "Sairey Gamps" and by the new occupation of monthly nurses who were willing to provide a month of postpartum domestic help and nursing under physicians' supervision. As a result, independent British midwives were in danger of extinction by the latter part of the nineteenth century. Nurses, on the other hand, whose position was clearly subordinate to physicians and whose previously negative public image had been greatly enhanced by the work of Florence Nightingale, were on the ascent.

Nightingale's subsequent attempt to upgrade the training and status of midwives in the 1860s was not as successful. She envisioned a two-tiered system of "midwifery nurses" with six months of training who could attend normal labor of the poor and "physician accoucheuses" with at least two years of training who could attend all cases. The model midwifery nurse program that she found closed after six years due to the sporadic outbreaks of puerperal fever common to all contemporary hospitals.

Nightingale's midwifery nurse program failed but her involvement lent new respectability to the declining occupation. Toward the end of the century midwifery began attracting unmarried, educated gentlewomen motivated by both humanitarian concerns and the need for income in a society with few opportunities for single women; midwives were expected and in some areas required to be unmarried until recent decades. Some of these more educated women joined to form the Midwives Institute (also known as the Matron's Aid Society), the precursor to the Royal College of Midwives.

Members of the Midwives Institute voluntarily embraced a position subordinate to male childbirth attendants to win their support for a midwifery registration system. For example, members took examinations offered by the Obstetrical Society even though the government repeatedly refused the society's request to require midwives to take them. Members also adhered to the restrictions proposed by the Obstetrical Society and attended mainly the natural labors of poor women. Members were willing to accept a medical man to represent their interests on a proposed midwives' regulatory board composed of physicians. Members were even willing to be subjected to a demeaning system of annual licensure by local authorities who could revoke a license, not only for professional misconduct, but also for other undefined misconduct in private life. Middle-class midwives were willing to accept subordination because they were more concerned with improving the maternity care of the poor than with enhancing the status of midwifery. From their first attempt in 1890 until they succeeded in 1902, the middle-class midwives' organization lobbied for legislation designed by physicians that would put them under medical control.

Donnison (1977:175) believes that if such repressive legislation had been adopted, midwifery would have disappeared completely in England as in the United States, given the uniform, centralized nature of government regulation. But such legislation was not adopted. Nineteenth-century British physicians were still too divided by social class to unite for a common goal. Nor did they all have the cultural authority that American physicians had gained by the twentieth century when the question of midwifery legislation arose here. Consequently, the traditional female occupation was preserved in Britain in spite of, or perhaps because of, the caustic, defamatory campaign waged, mainly by general practitioners, against midwives. The campaign culminated in 1901, when two women attended by midwives died after local physicians refused to provide emergency medical backup. Other general practitioners publicly endorsed their peers' actions as a means of eradicating midwives. This extremist position ignored public horror at the incident, increasing government concern about the falling birth rate in the face of defense needs and growing support for midwives' registration among influential, philanthropic, society women, including some wives of members of Parliament.

Under the guidance of members of the Home Office, the Local Government Board, and the Privy Council Office, the Midwives Institute successfully proposed a less repressive bill in 1902. This bill required only that the state-registered midwives notify local authorities of their intention to practice rather than submit to an annual licensure review. Moreover, the bill proposed that the Privy Council, rather than physicians, determine the composition of the Midwives

Board and have final say on its rules. This gave the midwives' regulatory board the same independence possessed by the physicians' board instead of giving the physicians' board control as had been proposed previously. Although midwives were not allowed to represent themselves on the regulatory board, they were given a specific representative. Another favorable change was the addition of two representatives from nursing organizations to the board. The divisive issue of prohibiting unqualified midwives from practicing was resolved with a compromise that gave existing "bona fide" midwives eight years to become qualified before being subject to prosecution.

The loss of annual local licensure control and complete regulatory authority over midwives was a blow to those physicians who hoped to eliminate midwives through hostile licensure. The act ensured a niche for midwives in Britain's health care system. Yet midwives did not gain the autonomy of self-regulation—the mark of a true profession. Unlike dentists, nurses, and most other health care professionals, midwives were to be supervised by physicians rather than by other midwives and their board would have a majority of physicians rather than peers.

These structural aspects of the act ensured that physicians could assume greater power over midwives. Nevertheless, in the early years some general practitioners tried to undermine the act by refusing to provide backup, ostensibly because of uncertainty about collecting their fees. Another act was passed in 1918 that put financial responsibility in the hands of the local supervising authorities when a patient could not pay. Donnison (177:185) believes that this was the turning point which improved relations between midwives and general practitioners. This act, combined with the earlier National Insurance Act of 1911, which covered the medical costs of the most indigent, left general practitioners less financially vulnerable and in need of routine maternity cases. As a result, they no longer needed to respond to midwives as competitors.

Midwifery in a Social Welfare State and the Transition to Hospital
As Britain continued to move toward a social welfare society, midwives increasingly worked as salaried or subsidized employees of clinics and hospital out-patient departments. Another act in 1936 required local health authorities to hire domiciliary midwives to con-

duct home births and to assist general practitioners attending home deliveries. The salaries were sufficient to make practice as an employee more attractive than independent practice to most midwives. The resulting bureaucratic organization also facilitated the upgrading of training requirements and the expansion of midwifery duties, further enhancing the public's image of midwives. In retrospect, some currently practicing midwives consider this period the golden era of British midwifery, although the hours were long, the pay low, and the practice settings uncomfortable and difficult. Midwives had public respect, alternatives in working situations, and a fair amount of independence in managing labor and delivery. They were backed up by general practitioners and a "flying squad" ambulance service.

This golden era did not last long. The structural changes in Britain's health care system and society at large led to the establishment of the National Health Service (NHS) in 1946. This program provided free, comprehensive health care, including the services of midwives, to all Britons. Ultimately, this program redefined midwifery.

The immediate effect of the NHS was to discourage the dwindling number of independent, fee-for-service, midwives in Britain. These women could not compete with the free care provided by the government. The ultimate impact of the NHS on the occupational territory of midwives was more far reaching. The NHS not only removed the cost differential between midwives and physicians but also removed the economic barrier that had kept many high risk, low-income mothers out of hospitals. In addition, the program paid general practitioners for obstetric cases whether or not they attended the deliveries. The latter provision created a resurgence of interest in routine prenatal care among general practitioners.

Government support for such a development had been building over the previous decade, in response to concerns about maternal mortality. As expected, the original Midwives' Act had reduced maternal mortality because midwives' new training enabled them to recognize complications and expeditiously transfer difficult cases to physicians. Nevertheless, after an initial decline in maternal mortality, the rate began to rise regardless of increasingly higher transfer rates (Donnison, 1977:187–90). Even more troublesome was the higher mortality among the more affluent, who were more likely to engage general practitioners. Ministry of Health investigations in the

1930s blamed the problem on general practitioners' continued use of unregistered midwives as assistants, the lack of emphasis on prenatal care, and the "meddlesome midwifery" of general practitioners inadequately trained to conduct obstetric operations in the septic conditions of working-class homes.[3] The ministry recommended that registered midwives replace unregistered midwives, that more general practitioners and midwives provide prenatal care, and that abnormal cases be attended in hospitals. The 1936 act helped to eliminate unregistered midwives, and the establishment of the NHS a decade later overcame the financial obstacles to prenatal care and hospital birth among the lower classes.

By 1958, 64 percent of births in Britain took place in hospitals (Ministry of Health, 1959). Twelve years later, the government-sponsored Peel Report found that the proportion of hospital births had mushroomed to 86 percent (Department of Health and Social Security, 1970). The report argued that one-fourth of the women who passed an initial screening and planned to deliver at home eventually required hospital care, and that a subgroup of them, who had to be admitted, experienced a higher perinatal mortality rate. These data led the committee to recommend building facilities that would promote 100 percent hospital deliveries. The rate now stands at 99 percent.

Incorporation with Nursing

The move into hospitals did not take childbirth out of the hands of midwives. Instead, midwives followed childbirth into hospitals. Eighty-one percent of the more than 20,000 midwives currently employed by the NHS work in hospitals (Macfarlane and Mugford, 1984:207–12).[4] The remainder work as community midwives providing mostly prenatal and postpartum care in homes, clinics, and physicians' offices. Midwives are still the senior persons present at about 76 percent of all births.

These statistics could be interpreted as evidence that midwifery is thriving in Britain. A closer examination tells a different story. As a

---

3. The death rate declined rapidly once antibiotics were adopted.

4. Fewer than 20 work as independent, fee-for-service, domiciliary midwives outside the NHS (personal communications).

result of the combined effects of the lack of professional autonomy inherent in the Midwives' Act, the bureaucratic structure of the NHS, and the hospital policy of the Peel Report, British midwives no longer control normal maternity care. Instead, the division of labor in hospitals has reduced midwives to assembly-line workers, while obstetrical consultants control the line.

Pregnant women's first contact with maternity care is now with their general practitioners rather than with domiciliary, community midwives as in the first half of the century. As a result, physicians, rather than midwives, generally confirm the pregnancy and arrange where and with whom the woman will deliver.

Midwives typically are involved in prenatal care only as part of hospital clinics' or general practitioners' staff. In these circumstances the midwives' role is largely limited to the nursing tasks of testing urine, checking blood pressure and weight, performing clerical duties, and chaperoning clients from room to room. A national survey in 1979 found that most midwives conduct prenatal abdominal examinations. However, 96 percent of hospital midwives and 86 percent of community midwives report that their examinations are repeated by a physician (Robinson et al., 1983:90, 115). Moreover, two-thirds of the midwives report that health visitors (an occupation similar to public health nurses in the United States) provide all or the majority of childbirth education where they work (Robinson et al., 1983:119).

Once in labor, most British women are attended by midwives. There is, however, a discrepancy between physicians and midwives about the role that midwives play in labor and delivery. Eighty-two percent of the midwives surveyed by Robinson and associates report that they manage all normal labors and call physicians only if they need assistance (1983:149). In contrast, only 46 percent of physicians believe this to be the case (p. 153). Similarly, the majority of midwives report that they decide when to conduct vaginal examinations, rupture membranes, and give analgesics in normal labors, whereas significantly fewer physicians believe that midwives have so much control (pp. 155, 163). Both acknowledge that fewer than 10 percent of midwives suture episiotomies or small tears (p. 169).

As is true for the prenatal period, the vast majority of midwives (85 percent) report that physicians repeat their postnatal examinations

(Robinson et al., 1983:218). The same proportion also states that physicians always decide when women are ready for discharge, even if midwives provided most, if not all, of the individuals' care (p. 222).

Although British midwives are involved in all phases of maternity care, there is little continuity of care. The midwife who attends a woman in labor is not likely to be the same midwife whom she met in a prenatal clinic or in her general practitioners' office. Neither is this midwife likely to attend her in the hospital after she gives birth, nor in the 10 days of statutorily required home visits by a community midwife after discharge. Typical of the treatment in a bureaucratic organization, hospital maternity care is fragmented by function and by standard work shifts. From the patients' viewpoint, integrated, efficient management now substitutes for personal continuity of care.

The repercussions for midwives are also serious. Once individual midwives specialize in certain areas, their skills in other areas may atrophy. This diminution of skills threatens the integrity of the occupation as a whole. Specialization and fixed work hours also mean that midwives rarely see the results of their actions and cannot evaluate their techniques. This fragmentation reinforces physicians' claim to management authority in normal as well as abnormal labor and delivery. As a result, most hospitals now have standard policies that direct midwives' actions on such procedures as the administration of drugs and use of fetal monitoring. With each new policy or standing order, a little more occupational territory is lost and the medicalization of childbirth grows.

As in the United States, the trend is toward the routine, active, medical management of childbirth. Midwives have become assistants in this process. Fetal monitoring is now standard in large teaching hospitals and is diffusing into smaller hospitals. Episiotomy has crossed the boundary between an abnormal and a normal procedure and is now performed in 53 percent of all vaginal births (Macfarlane and Mugford, 1984). The 7 percent cesarean section rate, although low by American standards, has been rising and inductions now stand at 36 percent after jumping from 15 percent in 1965 to 41 percent in 1975. The latest decline in inductions came after a study found no measurable benefits in fetal outcomes (Chalmers et al., 1978) but may simply reflect the increase in cesarean sections (Macfarlane, personal communication).

The distinct identity of British midwives is now in jeopardy. Since the turn of the century, most have trained first as nurses. In addition, many nurses who have little interest in working as midwives obtain the additional midwifery "qualification" to further their career goals in nursing administration, further diluting the occupation's identity.

In the past, the influence of nursing has been constrained by a sizable minority of midwives who came from "direct entry" programs for non-nurses. These women have a stronger identification as independent practitioners than do those with a nursing background. The number of such women is declining rapidly, however. Government policy has resulted in the virtual elimination of direct entry programs in recent years. As of 1985, only one program was accepting new students in England and no programs remained in Scotland, Wales, and Northern Ireland. The government also reduced the community experience in midwifery training programs from six to three months. As a result almost all midwifery training now is conducted in settings under direct medical control. These changes were capped with the passage of a bill in 1979 that combined the regulation of nurses, health visitors, and midwives, further eroding the independent identity of midwifery as an occupation.

Resistance to the diminished role of midwives and increased medicalization of childbirth began with consumer groups such as the Association for Improvements in Maternity Service, the National Childbirth Trust, the Society for Support of Home Confinements, and Birthrights, rather than with the Royal College of Midwives (Reid, 1984). A group of ten student midwives and one practicing midwife, stimulated by the growing consumer and feminist movements and the inaction of the Royal College, formed the Association of Radical Midwives (ARM) in 1976. The group has used the media to call attention to the continued erosion of midwifery and the medicalization of childbirth. By 1985 the association had about 500 British midwife members and had attracted more than 400 midwives to its last two conventions.

In spite of the growth of ARM most midwives appear unconcerned by recent changes. In a survey that we conducted in 1985 nearly half of the respondents said that working conditions are better now than they were 30 years ago.[5] Only 14 percent felt that they have become

---

5. Eighty percent of the 100 midwives working in one health district in southern England responded to our mail-back questionnaire.

little more than obstetric nurses, and fewer than half would like to see a revival of direct entry midwifery training programs. Very few expressed any qualms about gaps in their training; 90 percent felt that they had been adequately trained to handle normal childbirth and 81 percent felt capable of handling abnormal cases in emergencies. They appeared to be more concerned about the effects of cuts in the NHS and staff shortages on the role and position of midwives than about redefinitions of their role through government policy. Sixty-five percent felt that the interests of midwives were well represented by the Royal College of Midwives.

To say that many British midwives fail to appreciate the consequences of past policy changes for the future of midwifery does not mean that they are content with their current role. Ninety-four percent would like to see more clinics in which midwives would hold full responsibility for prenatal care. Eighty percent want responsibility for discharging women after normal childbirth. Slightly more than half would like more flexible work hours so that they could deliver mothers whom they attend in labor rather than providing fragmented care across shifts, and 37 percent would like to attend more home births. Whether they realize it or not, those midwives who are willing to accept greater responsibility, to give up the convenience of standardized work hours to provide personal continuity of care, and to function more independently as home birth attendants are seeking to regain their occupational territory.

AUSTRALIA

The Convict Era

The evolution of midwifery in Australia, as in the United States, is an outgrowth of the British experience, but at a later point in time. The western development of Australia did not begin until the American Revolutionary War deprived Britain of a place to transport the burgeoning number of convicts who could no longer be contained in its prisons. The ill-provisioned First Fleet of 11 ships arrived in Australia in 1788, with 188 convict women and 33 marine wives among the 1350 on board. Within a week, the first British baby was born in Australia.[6]

6. The discussion of the history of midwifery in Australia is based on the more

Historical records do not indicate whether anyone on the ships, including the ships' surgeons, had training in midwifery. Neither is there evidence that experienced midwives arrived with other early fleets. Yet the need was acute. In the first 50 years more than 11,000 women were transported to Australia to redress the imbalance of sexes in the penal colony. These convicts were joined by families of free settlers attracted by the government's promotion of opportunities in the new colony.

A Female Factory, established by the Governor to separate the sexes and provide employment for convict women, became the first maternity institution. Convict women, who worked as domestic servants for free settlers and military men, were sent to the factory if they became pregnant. Conditions there were bleak. The women and their children slept on the floor of the two workrooms; many had no blankets. They assisted one another when their time came.

Conditions were not that much better for most free settlers, who typically lived in tents and small huts. Those living outside settlements were attended only by their husbands or aboriginal women, unless another white woman lived nearby. Those in settlements, along with married convicts, did what they could for one another and called a surgeon in emergencies. How experienced the surgeons were in maternity care and what tools were available to them is open to question. In one notorious case in 1804 a surgeon was court-martialed because he did not respond when called, claiming that no forceps were available.

The inexperience of childbirth attendants was aggravated by nonexistent prenatal care, alcohol consumption, poor diet, venereal disease, unsanitary and damp conditions, and puerperal infection. As a result, maternal mortality was extremely high among both convict and free women. Infant mortality was also high, particularly among those born at the Female Factory. Babies who survived birth faced poor environmental conditions and early weaning. Many were abandoned since few jobs were available to single mothers. Single convicts who wanted to keep their children had to board them out to Baby Farms, where the mortality rate was appalling.

---

detailed account by Adcock et al. (1984) and brief overviews of Victoria, Tasmania, South Australia, New South Wales, and Western Australia by the Western Australian Branch of the National Midwives Association of Australia (1984). No information was available for Queensland in these reports.

In spite of the harsh conditions, fertility remained high into the nineteenth century. A few women gained reputations during these years as "fingersmiths," the convict slang for midwives. Two were listed on the 1806 roll, while another was appointed to the hospital facility in 1812. By 1820 a convict was employed as a resident midwife at the Female Factory, and a committee chaired by the governor's wife was established to assist poor, married women during their confinement in their own homes. In the same year a second Female Factory was established in the growing Hobart settlement. Convict women from this factory provided a lay midwifery service to the poor women of the area. They were joined in 1824 by a midwife with a diploma from Edinburgh who opened a private service for the more affluent. She was probably the first formally trained midwife in Australia.

The transportation of convicts ended in 1868. The convict hospitals were turned over to local authorities and the Female Factories were closed. As a result, all midwifery moved into homes, however humble.

Pioneer Expansion
Australia was radically transformed over the next 50 years. The success of the wool trade and the discovery of gold in 1851 lured huge numbers of immigrants. The population of Australia more than tripled between 1861 and 1901 (Mitchell, 1983). With the growth of population came a major transformation in social and economic organization. Australia changed from a struggling penal colony with little basic infrastructure in housing, transportation, health care, education, and industry to a rapidly developing nation by 1901.

The exponential population growth was caused not only by the arrival of immigrants but also by the children these typically young adults bore once in Australia. The number of midwives grew in response through immigration and home-grown experience, as did the number of physicians.

Unlike in the United States, most of these physicians were trained in Britain.[7] They emigrated to Australia in search of better economic

7. The discussion of the history of physicians and the subordination of midwives in Victoria from 1880 to 1930 draws on the excellent analysis of Willis (1983).

prospects. The nineteenth-century expansion of Australia had coincided with the breakdown of the guild system in Britain and the expansion of middle-class medical practitioners there. The resulting competition had made building a practice in Britain increasingly difficult for a new physician without family ties. Australia offered these physicians less competition and a less rigid social structure, as well as inexpensive pastoral leases and, after 1850, gold. In contrast, the United States had long since declined as a destination for British physicians. The market here was oversaturated; there were already 42 medical schools in the United States by 1850 (Starr, 1982:42), while Australia did not open its first until 1862 and it graduated too few to have any impact on the profession until the twentieth century (Willis, 1983:55).

The British middle-class background of most nineteenth-century Australian physicians had significant repercussions on the fate of midwifery in that country. As in the United States, these physicians had been trained in a system which increasingly expected physicians rather than midwives to attend births among the affluent. They came to Australia with few reservations about practicing obstetrics. Consequently, the first Australian medical school from its inception required training in childbirth, more than two decades before elite physicians ended their opposition to its inclusion in British medical curricula.

Following the British model, Australian physicians during the second half of the century helped to establish lying-in hospitals to gain clinical experience for medical students and to serve the poor. Training programs for Ladies Monthly Nurses were initiated at the Melbourne and Sydney hospitals in the 1860s to provide assistants for physicians who attended the home births of wealthy "squatters' " wives. To the consternation of many physicians, some of the monthly nurses began independent practices as midwives. Also during this period some midwives began to take women into their own residences, establishing private maternity hospitals. One mother-daughter team in New South Wales delivered 3,000 babies between 1870 and 1948.

These developments angered many physicians who, like their middle-class American counterparts, questioned "whether the practice of obstetrics should be permitted to women at all" (excerpt from an

Australian Medical Journal editorial quoted in Willis, 1983:104). The geographic and economic realities of Australia, however, combined with continuing close ties to Britain, undermined this opposition. While the early settlements had become more civilized, pioneers continued to press into the vast outback in search of good land and minerals, far from any medical services. The wealth created by agriculture and mining was concentrated in relatively few hands, and many Australians continued to live in dire poverty. These women could not afford physicians' services, and nurses had to be sent out of hospitals to assist many maternity cases. An example of such a case involved a woman whose "husband [was] laid up with rheumatic fever, [and who had] seven children, [with] only one blanket between them" (quoted in Adcock et al., 1984:36). The few lying-in hospitals could not accommodate all who needed their services. The one in Adelaide, for example, would take only married women until 1917. Moreover, puerperal sepsis was still a constant threat in hospital childbirth. As public concern for the plight of poor pregnant women grew, physicians accepted the need for trained midwives to work "outdoors," as domiciliary midwifery was called then, as well as in lying-in hospitals.

In 1870, the Sydney maternity hospital appointed a woman trained by Nightingale to supervise the introduction of Nightingale's midwifery training there. A midwifery course was begun at the Melbourne hospital in 1888 and turned into a nurse-midwifery program in 1893. A few other nurse-midwifery training programs also were begun at the end of the century. One in Sydney permitted experienced midwives who had not received formal training to attend lectures and take examinations. A precedent was established by these programs for physicians to provide lectures in midwifery while nurses and nurse-midwives provided training in nursing and domestic work. In 1899 the Melbourne hospital adopted a policy of hiring only midwives with general nurse training for its midwifery department. Like the other maternity hospitals, it opened an outdoor District Nursing Service as well to provide pregnant women with an alternative to untrained nonnurse-midwives.

As these developments reveal, the close ties to Britain and Australia's geographic and economic constraints ensured that physician opposition would not end midwifery in Australia, as it largely had in the United States. The early introduction of Nightingale's nurse-midwifery model also ensured the eventual subordination of midwifery and incorporation with nursing, as in Britain. Unlike Britain, however, the fragmented control of health care in the Federation of Australian States and the sparsely settled, vast, rural areas continued to provide an opportunity for functionally autonomous nurse-midwives for some time.

Twentieth-Century Subordination

Although the number of Australian training programs was growing at the turn of the century, only 10 percent of the approximately 2,000 midwives practicing at that time had formal training. The high cost of obtaining training—as much as 50 pounds—undoubtedly deterred many women. Others were hesitant to enter programs that took from six to twelve months and required students to work twelve or more hours a day, seven days a week, carrying patients up stairs, scrubbing floors and furniture, and sometimes doing cooking and laundry, as well as attending lectures and caring for patients. They had to do this while maintaining a neat and clean ankle-length uniform with a starched apron, collar, cuffs, and cap. Once trained, they could go into private practice or join the District Nursing Branch of a hospital and deliver babies, often in squalid conditions. Nevertheless, the Sydney facility had a six-month waiting list.

The demand for midwives generally exceeded the supply despite some decline in the Australian birth rate. Willis (1983:108) reports that the Victorian state government pressured the Melbourne hospital to give some formal midwifery training to practicing nonnurses to fill the gap. Physicians and nurses successfully opposed this change, which might have led to a permanent independent occupation of midwifery.

The enactment of midwifery registration in 1902 in Great Britain stimulated debate about whether a similar act should be passed in Australia. Besides the issue of untrained practitioners, there was also worry about the wide variation in training standards. Tasmania had already established a midwives' register in 1901 but the screening criteria appear to have been minimal until 1911, the same year that Western Australia introduced a very liberal registration program.

Some physicians supported the registration and regulation of midwives and repeatedly introduced state legislation to that effect. These efforts were blocked by the far more numerous physicians who opposed the legislation, despite their use of untrained women as assistants, and loudly voiced concerns about the qualifications of independent midwives. Others opposed to midwifery regulation felt that it would be impossible to provide enough trained practitioners to serve the vast rural areas. This problem later prevented the Victorian state government from following the Medical Association's recommendation that the 1908 Medical Registration Act ban "unqualified" practice. The Victorian Trained Nurses Association also came out strongly against midwifery registration out of fear that a separate occupation of midwifery would weaken their argument for the registration of nurses. The repeated failures to regulate midwives in the more populated states of New South Wales and Victoria led the Australian Trained Nurses Association to set up voluntary programs.

A Midwives Act was finally passed in Victoria in 1915. The subordinating nature of the act is evident. Midwives were refused the right to attend abnormal cases and to sue for nonpayment. Their regulatory board of three included two physicians and no midwives, and, unlike physicians, they were required to pay an annual registration fee to practice, be of good character, and bathe in disinfectant (Willis, 1983:113–15). In recognition of the shortage of trained nurse-midwives, bona fide midwives were allowed to register and made up 83 percent of the 700 names on the first register. Unregistered midwives were prevented from receiving payment for attending childbirth.

Incorporation with Nursing and the Transition to Hospital
Although the 1915 act placed Victorian midwives under the control of physicians, it did maintain midwifery's independence from nursing. This independence ended in 1928, when the Midwives Board was abolished and control vested in the Nurses Registration Board, as had already occurred in South Australia in 1920. Control of midwifery also was given to Nursing Boards in New South Wales in 1926 and in Western Australia in 1944. Like the Midwifery Boards before them, these Nursing Boards were dominated in their early days by physicians.

Untrained non-nurse-midwives were encouraged to attend classes under the new regulations. Also, beginning in the late 1920s, health authorities in New South Wales used nurse inspectors to supervise

the work of midwives and improve the education of untrained midwives. By 1930, 90 percent of the practicing midwives in New South
Wales were registered. The transition was nearly over; Australian
midwives had been both subordinated to physicians and incorporated with nurses. As in Britain the incorporation was so complete that it
became customary for nurses who hoped to advance their career to
take a second "qualification" in midwifery, even though few intended a career in that field.

While physicians, nurses, and midwives debated the pros and cons
of midwifery regulation, the federal government had other concerns. The growth of Australia's capitalistic economy was believed to
depend on the quantity and health of its labor force (Willis,
1983:109–10). Yet immigration was erratic, the birth rate was declining, and maternal and infant mortality were still high. In contrast,
Australia's Asian neighbors were experiencing rapid population
growth, raising concerns about defense. These forces led to a "popu-
late or perish" ethos, in which maternal and child welfare became a
national priority.

Much of the blame for high mortality was directed by physicians at
independent midwives, as in the United States. Unlike the more
laissez-faire reaction in the United States and preempting eventual
developments in Britain, the Baby Bonus, a maternity allowance for
all white women regardless of need, was established in 1912 to encourage them to have more children and subsidize the cost of obtaining trained assistance at childbirth. Physicians opposed the program,
claiming that "the medical practitioner is proverbially a bad business
man, but the half trained or wholly untrained midwife is as keen as
any shark . . . [and they will] lure prospective mothers to engage
their services" (quoted in Willis, 1983:112). The result was exactly the
opposite: the proportion of births attended solely by midwives was
halved in the following decade as the allowance made birthing the
less affluent more attractive to physicians. By 1936 about 80 percent
of births in Sydney had a doctor supervising or attending. This shift,
however, did not reduce maternal and infant mortality significantly.
That change awaited the medical profession's slow acceptance of the
need for antisepsis, the development of prenatal care, and the introduction of antibiotics.

While physicians were taking over childbirth in urban areas, mid-

wives still played the major role in rural areas. In 1911 a Bush Nursing Association was founded in New South Wales to provide trained
nurse-midwives as an alternative to the mostly untrained local midwives. By 1923 they had established 28 centers in remote areas. Similar associations were set up in other states. With the development of
air transport, a Flying Doctor Service was developed to back up the
nurse-midwives who were often the only source of trained health
care in these isolated areas. The outcomes of childbirth in the bush
hospitals were good and the women who ran these centers received
much public respect for their dedication and service.

The bush hospitals, along with the private cottage hospitals run by
midwives, offered midwives considerable autonomy in their personal
practice, even though the occupation as a whole was structurally
subordinate to physicians and incorporated within nursing. These
small facilities fell on hard times in the Depression, however, forcing
some to close. More closed during the war due to staffing shortages
and after the war due to lack of the more advanced medical technology which was increasingly considered necessary. Others grew
into larger hospitals. The gradual decline of these small facilities
reduced the opportunities for an independent midwifery practice.

Financial need forced many middle-class women to go to hospitals
for childbirth during the Depression. They were joined by upper-
class women, attended by their general practitioners, as puerperal
fever was brought under control. By 1950 almost 100 percent of
babies in New South Wales and Victoria were born in hospitals—two
decades before this rate was reached in Great Britain. The difference
points to the important role played by the network of small bush and
private cottage hospitals in Australia. There were so few home births
that the District Nursing Service in Victoria discontinued its domiciliary service in 1951 and focused on its new role of supplying postpartum visiting nurses.

In spite of the early transition to hospital, midwives continued to
deliver low risk uninsured working- and middle-class women during
the postwar baby boom. They constitued about 75 percent of all
maternity patients (Hayes, personal communication, 1984). Increasingly, however, midwives delivered these women under physician supervision as salaried employees of large public hospitals
rather than as independent practitioners. They also attended the
labors of physicians' private patients in hospitals and cared for them

during their ten- to eleven-day postpartum stay. Until recently, all Australian states legally required that every woman be attended by a midwife during childbirth.

Few midwives opposed working in hospitals and the resulting fragmentation of care. Industrial unions, first formed by nurses in the 1930s, had fought successfully for many improvements in hospital working conditions including pay during training, shorter work hours, elimination of the marriage restriction, limitation of work duties, and better pay. Like British midwives, they found hospital work more attractive than the still-legal alternative of domiciliary practice. The demand for home birth midwives was low; the population increasingly viewed childbirth as a medical event requiring pain-relief medication and the active obstetrical management available only in hospitals.

As in the United States, the number of obstetricians in private practice multiplied rapidly in the 1960s and 1970s, even though the national birth rate plummeted in 1971. These specialists have encroached on the territory of both general practitioners and midwives, and the proportion of births delivered by midwives and general practitioners in the large hospitals has declined.

Midwifery under a National Health Insurance System
The erosion of midwives' responsibilities has gained impetus since the 1970s from the federal government's subsidy of health insurance and nationalization of hospital costs. While the extent of coverage provided by the health insurance subsidy has been highly controversial and has changed several times, the new policies encourage women to use private obstetricians rather than midwife-staffed hospital clinics for prenatal care. The policies also make it possible for every woman to have a physician at her delivery if she wants. At the same time and as in other countries, the length of hospital stay has declined to two or three days, reducing the midwives' postpartum role.

Midwives' position has eroded in other ways as well. The last direct entry program ended in 1971. The number of births observed and delivered in training have been reduced. The recent trend toward regionalization of health care delivery has resulted in closing many small hospitals in which midwives managed maternity care. A controversial amendment was passed in Western Australia in 1983 that allows any nurse, whether qualified as a midwife or not, to work in maternity wards. Perhaps the most serious development is the new federal health care system, which does not allow a midwife to collect a fee for attending a home birth as an independent practitioner.

Home Birth

The last development is especially significant. At the same time that Australian midwives have seen their role in hospital maternity care shrink, public concern about excessive medicalization of childbirth and demand for natural childbirth have increased. As in the United States, this concern has led to a resurgence of home births. Between the mid-1970s and 1982 more than 5,000 women had planned home births, including the prime minister's daughter (Ligtermoet, 1983). In a national survey of recently trained nurse-midwives, 18 percent expressed a desire to have community experience in home birth added to their program (Barclay, 1984).

Interviews we conducted in 1984 with ten home birth midwives, including at least one from each Australian state and the Australian Capital Territory reveal numerous similarities and a few interesting differences in the home birth movement in Australia compared to the United States. The major difference is that no laws prevent registered midwives from attending home births although Victorian midwives must work under physician supervision. Neither do explicit laws prevent lay midwifery as long as there is no payment involved. Approximately half a dozen physicians attend home births in the largest cities using lay or nurse-midwives as assistants.

The participation of physicians and nurse-midwives does not mean that most physicians or nurses approve of home birth. Both the Royal Australian College of Obstetricians and Gynaecologists and the Royal Australian College of General Practitioners oppose home births (Carpenter, 1985). All home birth practitioners report encountering hostility from physicians, nurses, and nurse-midwives. One physician who used lay midwives as assistants and accepted women who would be classified as too high risk for home birth under Arizona's conservative criteria has since been deregistered in Victoria. Pressure from colleagues has compelled other physicians to stop doing home births.

As a result of the medical profession's official opposition to home birth, most home births are attended by midwives. Unlike in the

United States, however, most of these midwives are registered nurse-midwives. Their motivations for attending home births are the same as those of their American counterparts, although the career path of these nurse-midwives differs somewhat. Most intended to be general nurses but took their midwifery certificate because "it was the automatic thing to do," particularly if one wanted to improve one's job prospects or to travel. Several of those interviewed had worked or trained in England. Most of the rest have been abroad as well. All have practiced in hospital maternity wards. They became interested in home birth from a consumer perspective, as is common among American lay midwives, even though several have never had children.

The structure of their practice also differs somewhat from that of American lay midwives. Although legal, they cannot advertise directly and the cost of a professional listing in the phone book is prohibitive. Some were recruited by consumer home birth organizations that provide referrals and partial equipment. Others rely on word-of-mouth and referrals from physicians and health departments. Midwives in one state use birth kits provided by the local health department. The rest supplement their own equipment with equipment provided by their clients.

Unlike in the United States, most go to their client's homes for prenatal care and most attend births alone rather than in pairs or groups. In some Australian states no specific regulations direct independent nurse-midwives' screening criteria, guide their practices, or limit their clinical procedures. This may change: New South Wales was in the process of developing some regulations in 1985. Meanwhile, those who work without regulations use liberal screening criteria. In contrast, even in the absence of explicit rules, they are very conservative about procedures. Only rarely will midwives cut episiotomies or suture lacerations. The conservative use of common hospital midwifery procedures such as rupturing membranes and performing episiotomies stems from their philosophical commitment to natural childbirth for normal cases. The rarity of midwives who suture lacerations, on the other hand, results from their lack of training in this procedure.

All home birth midwives work with backup physicians. These physicians usually are involved more actively in prenatal care than is typical in the United States. Some of these physicians occasionally attend the births, perhaps because of their perceived ethical obligations in filing for their maternity care fee under the national insurance system, as well as their vulnerable professional position. Other midwives work more closely with physicians—sharing prenatal responsibilities, monitoring labors, and delivering babies only when the physicians do not arrive in time. Whether any of these physicians can take over care in the event of a hospital transfer depends on the local hospital's organization. No hospitals refuse transfer cases, but in some hospitals the staff take over care.

The new health care system makes no provision for reimbursing the fees of midwives who work as independent home birth practitioners or who assist physicians doing home births. Yet physicians involved in prenatal care receive a set fee for normal, uncomplicated maternity care whether they attend the birth or not. Some physicians who attend the births charge clients an additional amount above that allotted by the government for extra time involved in home birth. Midwives charge clients a flat, out-of-pocket fee of about A\$400 for prenatal, labor and delivery, and postpartum care. If their client has purchased a voluntary supplemental insurance policy that covers home health care, they can apply for reimbursement of about half a midwife's usual fee for home nursing care if they have a physician's written order. The midwives resent the implication of this circumvention:

> We are not paid as midwives. We're not recognized that we can catch babies and give care beforehand. We're only recognized as nurses who are underlings of doctors, because of our health system.

They are lobbying to have this situation changed.

NEW ZEALAND

Maternity care has a much shorter history in New Zealand than in the other countries considered. Prior to the Treaty of Waitangi in 1840, New Zealand was inhabited only by warring Polynesian tribes, sealers, whalers, timber traders, former and escaped Australian convicts, and missionaries. The treaty gave the British government the exclusive right to purchase land from the Maoris. This land was given to ex-soldiers and distributed by lottery to settlers. As a result, there was a large influx of population; 19,000 came between 1839 and 1843 alone. Gold brought 35,000 in 1863 and land grants attracted a steady stream of free migrants including some British middle-class physicians. Return migration was also high (Mitchell, 1983:145), but the population increased sufficiently by the latter part of the nineteenth century to make the establishment of private maternity homes for the more affluent an attractive option for some physicians. The rest continued to rely on lay midwives.

The Early Introduction of Regulation

A desire to increase the birth rate led New Zealand's Parliament to follow the lead of Great Britain and pass a Midwives Registration Act in 1904.[8] As in the mother country, it passed over physician opposition. This act established the first state-operated maternity hospital to train midwives and to provide maternity care for the poor and working class. A British-trained nurse-midwife set up and managed the program. Within two years, two other maternity hospitals with similar midwifery training programs had opened and land had been bought for a third.

The midwifery training programs took one year and allowed for direct entry of non-nurses. The one physician on staff was the medical superintendent, generally a woman, who was called only in problem cases. Midwives trained the students to practice independently and to assume full responsibility for normal births. As in Australia and Great Britain, nurses interested in furthering their career or travelling typically took midwifery training even though they did not intend to practice as midwives.

Incorporation with Nursing

Midwifery training changed radically in 1925 when Parliament set up a combined Nurses and Midwives Board. As in other countries, the joint regulation of nurses and midwives facilitated the incorporation of midwifery into nursing. Responding to physician complaints that the 20 births delivered and 30 observed by each student midwife deprived medical students of clinical experience, the board reduced

8. Information on the history of midwifery in New Zealand comes from Donley (1981, 1985a, 1985b).

the training period to six months and changed the focus of the program to producing mostly maternity nurses to work under physician supervision rather than as independent practitioners. The intake of direct entry midwifery students was reduced immediately by half.

About the same time, the Health Department contemplated a state-run maternity service staffed only by midwives. Physicians who felt that such a service would encroach on their private practices formed an Obstetrical Society in 1926 and successfully opposed the program. This association enabled physicians to lobby for their interests in a more effective way than could the unorganized midwives.

Midwifery in a Socialized Medical System

The Obstetrical Society proved particularly useful when a Commission of Enquiry into Maternity Services was set up in 1937. New Zealand was about to begin the first comprehensive socialized medical care system in the world and the government wanted to develop a formal policy on maternity care as part of this program. The commission acknowledged that practicing midwives were highly trained. Under the influence of the Obstetrical Society, however, it expressed concern that physicians were denied access to so many births occurring in public hospitals which could provide them needed training and practice. Members debated discontinuing all midwifery training and transferring the public maternity hospitals to the general hospital board. Members also considered the increased demand among women for "twilight sleep," which was only available at private, physician-run hospitals. In the end, the commission recommended retaining public maternity hospitals and midwifery training on a small scale but also recommended promoting hospital childbirth and admitting medical students into the public maternity hospitals.

When the socialized health care system began in 1938, home birth midwives were allowed to continue practicing under contract with the Department of Health. Unlike what was to come later in Great Britain and Australia, New Zealand midwives were paid by the government as independent practitioners on a fee-for-service basis. They could be paid, however, only for one prenatal visit, labor and delivery, and a maximum of 14 postpartum visits. This limitation put physicians, not midwives, in charge of prenatal care. By making physicians the initial care providers, the system encouraged women to use physicians for labor and delivery as well and to go to hospitals for birth.

Although the number of home birth midwives dwindled, a few continued to work under contract with the Department of Health. The Nurses Act of 1971, however, outlawed lay midwifery and took away midwives' right to attend clients independently. Clients now must have a backup physician who takes responsibility for their care. A 1983 Nurses Amendment Bill further diminished the status of midwives; it required that all future home birth midwives also be registered nurses and, like the recent legislation in Western Australia, allowed nurses without midwifery training to supervise hospital maternity care. As a result, Donley argues, the hospital "midwife is seen as having no more expertise than a nurse" (1985a:5).

This change in status has been facilitated by the continued erosion of midwifery training in New Zealand. Direct entry programs no longer exist. The original public maternity hospitals were transferred to Hospital Boards in the 1970s and only one still operates as an obstetric unit. The six-month hospital-based midwifery course ended in 1979. Under the leadership of the New Zealand Nurses Association, training moved into the technical schools, where the nursing component was augmented and the obstetric component reduced to between eight and twelve weeks, depending on the program. Many New Zealand nurses now go overseas to Australia or Great Britain to do a hospital-based midwifery program. Of the 171 midwives registered with the New Zealand Nursing Council in 1982, only 14 percent were trained in New Zealand. Although some of those trained abroad are immigrants, more than one-quarter took their nurse training in New Zealand before going abroad.

Home Birth

Just when home birth midwives had become a virtual anachronism in New Zealand, there was a rebirth of consumer interest. About 1,000 of the approximately 370,000 births that occurred in New Zealand between 1975 and 1981 were planned home births (New Zealand Home Birth Association, 1981). New Zealanders chose home birth for the same reasons as women elsewhere. The number of obstetrical specialists was growing, regionalization was closing the smaller hospitals staffed by general practitioners and midwives, and active management in the birth process was expanding. Interested consumers formed numerous local home birth associations beginning in 1978 (New Zealand Home Birth Association, 1982). These have since linked together in a national association. Another group called Save the Midwives was set up by consumers in response to the deterioration of midwives' status caused by the 1983 Nurses Amendment Bill. This group focuses on public education and political lobbying.

About 16 home birth midwives were practicing in the country in 1985. Although the number is small in comparison to the United States or even Australia, the population of New Zealand is only 3,295,000. Interviews conducted with 11 of these women scattered around the country reveal that, as in Australia, almost all trained first as nurses and only later became interested in midwifery. Several went to England or Scotland for midwifery training. Almost all have worked as hospital midwives; a few still do on a part-time basis. They began doing home births to provide a better birth experience than they felt was generally available, especially in large base hospitals where ruptured membranes, fetal monitors, pain-relief medication, episiotomies, and rigid feeding schedules had become routine. As one says, "I thought . . . if I can deliver babies in hospital bathrooms and trolleys and cars and things, I couldn't see why I couldn't really do it at home."

A few who started practicing in the mid-1970s initially encountered considerable hostility from medical practitioners. One described feeling like a "backstreet abortionist" when she transferred women, even though the Health Department paid her for each case. Now, however, they report feeling "actually quite respectable." In 1984 the outgoing minister of health for the National Party granted a small raise in their meager pay and a redistribution of 2 of their 14 postpartum visits to the prenatal period. The new Labour government even promised to expand the role of home birth midwives. But after a year in office no changes had been made.

The midwives collect a maximum of NZ $167 for three prenatal visits, labor and delivery, and twelve postpartum visits. Any additional visits are at their own expense. Even a midwife with a high volume practice of 50 to 60 births per year would be hardpressed to maintain a household on her earnings. Nevertheless, they cannot charge clients additional fees under the socialized medical care system. In some cases, the local home birth association collects donations and provides midwives with beepers, one of their largest expenses. Many admitted that they relied on an understanding husband for financial support and two of those interviewed lived in communal arrangements. For New Zealand midwives, low pay, not opposition from physicians and hospital nurse-midwives, presents the major obstacle to their practice.

All have at least several general practitioners who will give prenatal care and take responsibility for home births; some have as many as seven in their local area. Unlike in the mid-1970s, most general practitioners now try to come to the birth, although they need only to see the woman within 24 hours to collect their fee from the government. None of the midwives believes that physicians endure the inconvenience of coming to the birth for economic motives. Instead, they point to the opposition of obstetricians to home births and the structure of the health care system, which puts prenatal care "in the hands of the doctors. . . . They're the ones who put their heads on the chopping block when it comes to doing home births because they're the ones who are taking the legal responsibility." As a result, the physicians feel more secure if they are present. The midwives also say that most keep coming after they become familiar with midwives' skills both because they build a relationship with clients during prenatal care and because they begin to enjoy home births after attending a few. The midwives welcome their presence. Like the Australian home birth midwives, they work alone and occasionally need an extra pair of hands. They also believe that the exposure to natural childbirth has a positive influence on how the physicians treat their hospitalized maternity patients.

General practitioners' new willingness to cooperate with midwives stems from a growing recognition that their right to practice also is threatened by specialists. General practitioners are still responsible for more than half the 50,000 annual births in the country, but their participation in maternity care is declining. The move toward regionalization of maternity care, pushed by the Head of the Post Graduate School of Obstetrics, is aimed at phasing out general practitioners who "lack experience [in] managing abnormalities" and lack adequate facilities in the smaller hospitals to provide more than "aggregated domiciliary confinement" (quoted in Donley, 1985a:7). The elimination of maternity care in smaller hospitals will leave general practitioners with no place to attend births since specialists staff the central hospitals.

The home birth midwives who began practicing in the mid-1970s also report a major change in the attitude of hospital midwives toward them. One told about engaging in a "nasty argument" with hospital midwives concerning the refusal of the New Zealand Nurses Association to submit a position paper, written by the Midwives Section, to the select committee that was developing the 1983 Nurses Amendment. She argued that "somewhere along the line you have to make a decision as to what you really are and whether you're a nurse-midwife, which is merely an obstetrician's handmaiden, or whether you're a midwife, which is a practitioner in your own right." When the amendment undermined the position of hospital midwives as well, Donley (1985b:1) reports, "it politicized the hospital-based midwives as nothing else could have done." Like others, she reports (personal communication, 1985) that "I'm their long lost friend and they ask me to speak at seminars . . . and they're very supportive of home birth because they're finding out that we're the ones who have the consumer support. They haven't."

Donley's perceptions are supported by the results of a survey that we conducted in 1985 of all midwives working in the Waikato Health District hospitals.[9] Unlike the British midwives whom we surveyed, only 37 percent of the New Zealand midwives say that they were trained to conduct normal childbirth without a physicians' supervision and most of these had trained in Britain or Australia. Also unlike the British midwives, 60 percent feel that midwives have become little more than obstetric nurses in New Zealand.

In spite of the recognized reduction in the role of hospital midwives and widespread complaints of staff shortages and low pay,

9. Mail-back questionnaires were given to administrators of each hospital to distribute among hospital midwives working full and part time on all shifts. At the time of the survey, 76 midwives were employed in the base hospital and about 50 were employed in district hospitals. Some of these midwives, particularly those who work infrequently in response to staffing needs, did not receive a questionnaire, but not all administrators returned undistributed questionnaires as requested. The 86 completed questionnaires constitute two-thirds of all midwives estimated to be practicing.

three-quarters of the New Zealand midwives feel that working conditions have improved in the last 20 years. Only 29 percent, however, feel that the Nursing Council adequately represents their current interests. While less than one-quarter support a revival of midwifery training programs for non-nurses, 59 percent would like to see more rigorous screening of applicants for nurse-midwifery training on the basis of career plans. Sixty percent feel that midwives should be allowed to manage normal childbirth in the hospital without a physician's supervision. An even larger proportion, 75 percent, believe that maternity care would be improved if a midwife followed a mother through her prenatal, labor and delivery, and postpartum care rather than being assigned to only one of these tasks, and two-thirds would be willing to work "longer and less predictable hours" in order to deliver women whom they have attended in labor.

The greatest agreement among the hospital midwives concerns the medicalization of hospital childbirth. Eighty percent feel there is "too much medical and surgical intervention these days." This belief is linked to favorable attitudes toward home birth. Even though the majority acknowledge that "you can never really say who is a 'low risk' maternity patient until after the delivery" and "homes do not have the necessary technology for intervention when problems arise," most do not find these persuasive arguments against home birth. Only 24 percent agree that "home births are dangerous, unnecessary and should be discouraged." Although a quarter do not feel adequately trained in labor and delivery to attend home births, 43 percent would be willing to deliver a planned home birth in the future and 60 percent would be willing to assist a physician doing one. Their reasons for not attending home births at this time include low pay (75 percent), irregular work hours (67 percent), low demand by women (63 percent), lack of an adequate transfer system (54 percent), reluctance to take on so much responsibility (47 percent), and not knowing a physician willing to provide backup (42 percent).

THE CONVERGENT FATE OF MIDWIFERY IN ENGLISH-SPEAKING COUNTRIES

Although the four countries considered share common historical roots and a varying degree of continued cultural exchange, each has developed a different health care system reflecting its unique pattern of demographic, economic, social, and political development. Yet the fate of midwifery may ultimately be much the same.

Midwives virtually disappeared in the competitive free market of turn-of-the-century American medicine. As discussed in chapter 1, this occurred largely before modern medicine had much to offer and before the transition to hospital had taken place. The midwives' place was taken by general practitioners, who have since been replaced by obstetricians, assisted by staff nurses and residents who monitor the time-consuming labors. When physicians were in short supply in the 1960s, nurse-midwifery was expanded to service poor and rural populations.

In Great Britain, Australia, and New Zealand the competition for maternity care was never as great as in the United States. When the move to hospitals came, midwives went with the women, to service the working class and poor and monitor labor for the private patients of physicians. The timing of the shift to institutions varied. The transition came first in Australia, long before the incorporation of midwifery with nursing and the proliferation of obstetrical specialists. The transition came because the government's desire for population growth and the general impoverishment of the population led to the creation of numerous charitable institutions and the early introduction of a Baby Bonus. The change came next in New Zealand, where a similar concern for population growth led to the formation of maternity hospitals run originally by midwives, as envisioned by Nightingale. The move to hospitals happened last in Great Britain, where it awaited the removal of the financial barriers that had prevented poor and working-class women from visiting a general practitioner for prenatal care and having their babies in hospitals.

After the transition to hospital, the role of a midwife in each country depended largely on the location of the hospital, the degree to which midwifery was incorporated with nursing, and the availability of physicians. New Zealand led the others in establishing the joint regulation of nurses and midwives. The rigor of midwifery training began to decline immediately and direct entry programs were phased out to provide more training opportunities for physicians. The majority of New Zealand's hospital midwives now recognize that they function as little more than maternity nurses unless they work in the remaining rural hospitals.

In contrast to New Zealand, fragmented state control in Australia delayed the final incorporation of midwifery with nursing there. Even after control was accomplished in each state, Australian midwives who worked in rural areas continued to function autonomously because of a lack of physicians. But, as in New Zealand, the recent push for regionalization by the increasing number of obstetricians is driving out both general practitioners and functionally autonomous midwives. The requirements of training programs in several states have declined, and Australian hospital midwives are well on their way to becoming merely highly skilled maternity nurses.

British midwives are still confident of their training and role, and most (65 percent) believe that the Royal College of Midwives represents their interests effectively. Yet the college has not halted the reduction of community experience in their training programs or the closure of all except one direct entry program. Most important, in view of the experience of New Zealand and Australian midwives, it did not oppose the joint regulation of midwives and nurses introduced in 1979. As the small, but vocal, Association of Radical Midwives recognizes, while this legislation reduced physicians' legal domination of midwifery, it greatly increased the chances that British midwives too will become highly trained maternity nurses.

REFERENCES

Adcock, Winifred, Ursula Bayless, Marcetta Butler, Pamela Hayes, Hazel Woolston, and Patricia Sparrow. *With Courage and Devotion: A History of Midwifery in New South Wales*. Wamberal, Australia: Anvil, 1984.

Arney, William R. *Power and the Profession of Obstetrics*. Chicago: University of Chicago Press, 1982.

Barclay, Leslie. "An enquiry into midwives' perceptions of their training." *Australian Journal of Advanced Nursing* 1:11–24, 1984.

Carpenter, Hugh. "Domiciliary obstetrics." *Australian Family Physician* 14:207–14, March 1985.

Chalmers, Iain, M. E. Dauncey, E. R. Verrier-Jones, J. A. Dodge, and O. P. Gray. "Respiratory distress syndrome in infants of Cardiff residents during 1965–75." *British Medical Journal* 2:1119–21, 1978.

Department of Health and Social Security. *Domiciliary Midwifery and Maternity Bed Needs*. London: Her Majesty's Stationery Office, 1970.

Donley, Joan. "Midwifery in New Zealand," unpublished report. 1985[a].

Donley, Joan. *Report from New Zealand to Homebirth Australia Conference.* April 1985[b].

Donnison, Jean. *Midwives and Medical Men: History of Inter-Professional Rivalries and Women's Rights.* London: Heinemann, 1977.

Forbes, T. "The regulation of the English midwife in the 18th and 19th centuries." *Medical History* 15:352–62, 1971.

Hinds, Cora. "A place for the nurse-midwife." *International Nursing Review* 32:46–47, 1985.

Ligtermoet, Henny. *National Homebirth Figures, Natural Childbirth Newsletter.* 1983.

Macfarlane, Alison, and A. Mugford. *Birth Counts: Statistics of Pregnancy and Childbirth.* London: Her Majesty's Stationery Office, 1984.

Ministry of Health. *Report of the Maternity Services Committee.* London: Her Majesty's Stationery Office, 1959.

Mitchell, B. R. *International Historical Statistics: The Americas and Australia.* London: Macmillan Reference Books, 1983.

New Zealand Home Birth Association (Auckland Branch). *Newsletter,* No. 12, 1981.

New Zealand Home Birth Association. "Home birth in New Zealand today." *NAPSAC News* 7:19+, 1982.

Reid, Margaret. "From home birth to active birth: The British midwife." *Mothering* 30:70–74, 1984.

Robinson, Sarah, Josephine Golden, and Susan Bradly. *A Study of the Role and Responsibilities of the Midwife.* London: Department of Health and Social Security, 1983.

Starr, Paul. *The Social Transformation of American Medicine.* New York: Basic Books, 1982.

Western Australian Branch of the National Midwives Association of Australia. *History of Midwifery Practice in Australia and the Western Pacific Regions,* 20th Congress, International Confederation of Midwives. Sydney, 1984.

Willis, Evan. *Medical Dominance.* Sydney: Allen & Unwin, 1983.

CHAPTER 10

REBIRTH OR FALSE LABOR?
THE FUTURE OF MIDWIFERY
IN THE UNITED STATES

The modernization of health care, like the modernization of society in general, has been a process of increasing specialization of function. Health care has grown from a domestic task relegated primarily to women into a large-scale, bureaucratic, polynucleated corporate enterprise characterized by a highly differentiated division of labor (Starr, 1982:3, 421–49). In the course of growth, a succession of different occupations has evolved to provide care for women during childbirth. Each new occupation has established dominance by claiming to have more knowledge, experience, and techniques for identifying and managing complications than its predecessors. Each has brought a greater degree of medicalization to childbirth, and its forerunners have succumbed to incorporation, limitation, subordination, or exclusion. In contrast, modern independent midwives, the lay and nurse-midwives who practice out of hospitals, developed as a reaction to this medicalization trend.

THE RISE AND FALL OF CHILDBIRTH OCCUPATIONS

The emergence of traditional midwives was the beginning of specialization in maternity care. Their work was an extension of their gender role. As women, they were expected to help others at birth and often did as much housework as health care. They had only practical knowledge, acquired through experience, to use in assisting birth. The more experienced ones may have been able to manage breeches and small hemorrhages with manual techniques, but most could do little when serious complications developed.

Traditional midwives' inability to cope with more difficult problems created an opening for barber-surgeons to enter childbirth care. At first emergency childbirth assistance was only one of many diverse surgical tasks that they performed. When competition for work increased with the expansion of middle-class practitioners, however, some men began to deliver babies under normal circumstances as well, arguing that their surgical techniques made them better qualified than contemporary midwives.

The introduction of these man-midwives increased the differentiation of maternity care. They limited their function to delivery of the baby, leaving domestic chores to family members, servants, monthly nurses, or female assistant midwives. Aided by their status as men in a sexist culture, man-midwives successfully sought incorporation with physicians, access to theoretical information about childbirth physiology, and improved tools for intervention. They gained the patronage of the affluent and left the care of the poor to midwives.

The merger of man-midwives, barber-surgeons, and apothecaries with physicians made medicine the dominant authority on childbirth. In most developed countries, traditional midwives were replaced by midwives trained and regulated by physicians and limited to normal maternity care; these trained midwives were differentiated into nurse-midwives, who considered midwifery a specialized type of nursing, and direct-entry midwives, who viewed it as a distinct occupation. In contrast, in the United States traditional midwives were replaced directly by physicians.

Childbirth occupations became further differentiated as more physicians began to specialize in the unified fields of obstetrics and gynecology through residency programs, begun in the 1930s (Speert, 1980:82). Although general practitioners still attended most births in the United States and provided most prenatal and some childbirth care in other developed countries, obstetrician-gynecologists' extended training in the pathology of pregnancy and childbirth gave them greater authority. Their positions on medical school faculties and as hospital-based consultants allowed them to set standards for the far more numerous general practitioners.

The movement of birth into hospitals facilitated the incorporation of midwifery into nursing in those countries where it had remained a viable option. Most midwives willingly gave up private fee-for-service practice for the security and regular hours of salaried hospital work. Hospitals gradually phased out direct-entry training programs because they preferred the flexible staffing possibilities of nurse-midwives. Moreover, most hospital administrators believed that midwives needed nurse training as well.

Despite their increasing incorporation into nursing, the emergence of obstetricians, and the change in the locus of childbirth, midwives continued to be the primary attendants at childbirth in most countries for some years. Depending on the national availability of physicians, they attended either all normal births or only those of indigent and rural women. In both circumstances, they also provided primary care during labor and postpartum for physicians' patients.

In the United States, the short supply of physicians coupled with the lack of trained midwives to attend parturient women during the postwar baby boom led to a call for nurse-midwives. The new American occupation of certified nurse-midwives grew in response. Although they are trained to work autonomously, their practice is limited formally to attending normal childbirth under a physician's supervision. Until recently they also have been limited informally to serving indigent and rural women as salaried hospital or clinic staff.

The need for functionally autonomous midwives to provide care in rural areas and charity wards declined in the United States and elsewhere by the early 1970s. Most developed countries had become highly urbanized, and all had adopted programs for subsidizing the medical care costs of the poor. At the same time, the supply of physicians, particularly obstetrician-gynecologists, expanded while birth rates dropped precipitously. The end result has been intense competition for maternity work and an attempt by obstetrician-gynecologists to broaden their occupational territory to that of "women's primary physician" (Speert, 1980:248).

Obstetrician-gynecologists also have responded by pressing for additional limitations on the maternity care role of general practitioners and nurse-midwives. Using the authority derived from their greater expertise in diagnosing and managing complications, they have argued for regionalizing maternity care. This, they contend, will provide access to the more sophisticated and expensive technologies needed to actively manage labor and delivery and treat complications. The restructuring of regionalization entails closing the small maternity wards where nurse-midwives and general practitioners attend births in most Western developed countries. These closures are driving general practitioners out of maternity care because they have found it increasingly difficult, if not impossible, to gain obstetrical privileges at the large hospitals.

Obstetrician-gynecologists have sought to limit the role of nurse-midwives in other ways as well. They have broadened their definition of high risk to classify a larger proportion of maternity cases as in need of their services. In many countries, they also have supported reducing the clinical portion of midwifery training. These changes have pushed nurse-midwives toward the diminished role of a subordinated nursing assistant rather than a supervised limited practitioner capable of managing normal care (World Health Organization, 1985).

The division of labor in maternity care has changed again in recent years owing to the emergence of two new diametrically opposed occupations. The first, independent, fee-for-service lay and nurse-midwives, attend only low risk women in their homes or in free-standing birth centers. They assist women in natural childbirth unless complications develop. The second, perinatologists, are obstetricians who have been trained intensively in high risk maternity care. Neither occupation as yet attends a significant portion of births, but both are growing in numbers and clientele.

Perinatologists and independent midwives now encroach on the occupational territory of obstetrician-gynecologists much as obstetricians invaded the territory of general practitioners, who had previously penetrated the territory of trained midwives, who in turn took over most of the work of traditional midwives. Although obstetrician-gynecologists have mounted an aggressive defense against independent midwives, they appear not to recognize the threat posed by perinatologists. Gender discrimination may account for some of the difference in response, since perinatologists, like obstetricians, are overwhelmingly male. Perhaps more important, independent midwives, unlike perinatologists, emerged outside the fraternity of physicians. As a result, they are perceived as one of "them" rather than as one of "us." Perinatologists also do not compete directly for work in maternity care but instead depend on referrals from other physicians, mainly obstetrician-gynecologists. This lack of overt competition has led the latter to feel that they have nothing to fear from the growth of the former. Given the history of maternity care occupations, this sense of security may be groundless.

The current relationship between obstetrician-gynecologists and perinatologists parallels that of general practitioners and obstetricians earlier in this century. At that time obstetrical specialists were in short supply and worked mainly from referrals, like perinatologists today. As the number of specialists increased relative to the number of maternity cases, however, the specialists gradually broadened their targeted clientele to include low risk women. Those who seek to exclude general practitioners and trained midwives from maternity care argue that childbirth is never low risk.

The fact that obstetrician-gynecologists and perinatologists share a pathological view of childbirth and a common origin in medicine prevents the former from recognizing the threat that the latter pose to their continued dominance. Even if obstetricians recognized that their occupational territory was in jeopardy, they would be powerless to prevent the incursion of perinatologists. Perinatologists' claim to authority is based on their greater expertise in diagnosing and managing maternity complications. Obstetricians used this same argument to support their own invasion of maternity care and attack on general practitioners and modern midwives. They cannot retract this principle now. History suggests that if the relative number of perinatologists increases, they will seek a larger share of the maternity-care market and wrest dominance from obstetrician-gynecologists. The obstetrician-gynecologists in turn will push aggressively to eliminate competition from general practitioners and independent midwives while relying more on their gynecological work. Eventually the specialties of obstetrics and gynecology may divide into perinatologists and gynecologists. Alternatively, obstetrician-gynecologists may succeed in achieving authority as women's primary-care physicians.

CAN INDEPENDENT MIDWIFERY SURVIVE SUBORDINATION?

The future of independent midwives is more difficult to discern. DeVries argues that the licensure sought by modern American lay midwives ultimately will undermine them because all licensure "formalizes the dominance of physicians," and subordination is incompatible with occupational integrity (1985:140). Yet the history of midwifery on the European continent reveals that independent midwifery can flourish under physician supervision and legal limitation as long as it does not compete directly with medicine. While licensure restricted independent European midwives to normal childbirth and prohibited them from using instruments, it left most with considerable functional autonomy; countries with the most demanding training requirements for licensure—Holland, France, and Denmark—granted midwives the most individual latitude in their practice. Governmental control took the form of requirements for licensure, records, reports, and in some countries supervisory visits, but no country required screening of clients by physicians until recently (for a brief review of older European laws see White House Conference on Child Health and Protection, 1932:174–77).

In contrast, independent midwifery waned in the absence of regulation in the late nineteenth and early twentieth centuries in Britain and the United States. Independent midwifery in Britain was rescued only at the turn of the century with the adoption of centralized regulation that upgraded education and practice standards to those elsewhere in Europe.

The restrictive nature of the granny midwife laws subsequently introduced in the United States are often blamed for the demise of the traditional midwife here. The restrictions, however, were not much different from those in Europe. Neither did they differ significantly from those desired by modern independent midwives. The laws typically prohibited midwives from attending abnormal labors and using forceps, turning a mispositioned fetus in utero, or administering drugs other than antihemorrhagics (Foote, 1919:535–36).

The granny midwife laws contributed to the downfall of traditional midwifery not because of their restrictiveness but because of their lenience. Only a few states required formal training or an examination. Even fewer provided training programs beyond sporadic short courses (White House Conference on Child Health and Protection, 1932:178–95).

The leniency of granny midwife laws resulted from a compromise between American physicians who wanted to outlaw midwives and

those who wanted to upgrade their skills to improve the care provided to their impoverished clients. This debate is evident in the
report of the Obstetric Education Subcommittee of the 1932 White
House Conference on Child Health and Protection. The committee
noted the "very favorable maternal mortality" statistics of untrained
American midwives and the "remarkably low rates" of European
midwives and the few trained American midwives (1932:203). It acknowledged that "a large percentage of maternal mortality follows
operative interference . . . [by general practitioners who lack time to
be] . . . patient waiters by the bedside of those mothers who are normal" (217). The committee recommended that "at the present time,
the midwife is a necessity; and every effort should be made . . . to
improve her" (205), but warned against "overtraining" a group of
potential competitors. One member argued persuasively that the
"most dangerous midwife" from his perspective as a physician would
be "a very competent white woman" because she would not confine
herself to the indigent (212). To stem this threat, the committee
concluded that training should remain a local responsibility, that
schools be located "where they will not conflict with the obstetric
teaching work of medical schools" (206), and that "the ultimate solution . . . is in developing a sufficient number of physicians . . . well
trained in the fundamental principles of obstetrics" (205). Imple-
mentation of these recommendations left women with no way to
obtain good midwifery training, and left traditional midwives to
wither in their marginal practice among the rural poor while the
urban poor increasingly were attended by apprentice physicians.

The contrasting fate of midwives in the United States and Europe
provides evidence that subordination alone does not sound a death
knell for an occupation. For a subordinated occupation to flourish,
however, restrictions on practice must be balanced by a policy aimed
at giving it the same knowledge and skills within its limited area of
work as the dominant occupation. This will happen only if the subordinated occupation finds a niche where it will not compete directly
with the dominant occupation. It is these circumstances which allowed the trained midwives in early twentieth-century Europe, Australia, and New Zealand to function as loosely supervised limited
practitioners.

Although subordination does not eliminate a formerly autono-

mous occupation, it does have an effect. The more actively a dominant occupation participates in the training of a subordinated occupation, the more effectively it can socialize the latter to accept its
authority, perspective, and style of practice. As the case of unlicensed
American midwives demonstrates, this can happen even when an
occupation is not formally subordinated if it still must rely on the
dominant occupation for its knowledge base and for backup support
in the event of complications.

CAN INDEPENDENT MIDWIFERY SURVIVE INCORPORATION?

Incorporation with other groups poses a greater threat to the status
of an occupation than does subordination. Homeopaths, for example, could not survive incorporation with regular physicians, and
osteopaths now struggle to maintain their separate identity. Similarly, the early merging of midwifery with nursing in New Zealand
undermined the midwives' sense of competency by lowering their
training standards. The same process is underway in Australia and may
eventually occur in Britain and other European countries as well.

The erosion of occupational identity has been facilitated by policies
which minimize the obstetric component in general nursing and encourage nurses to obtain a midwifery qualification as a way of becoming "a complete nurse." The resulting large numbers of women
trained as midwives but lacking a commitment to the field dilute
midwifery as a specialized, skilled occupation.

The incorporation of midwifery with nursing in cultures derived
from Britain also has brought the formerly independent occupation
under the influence of the Nightingale philosophy of nursing. Nightingale believed that nurses should serve as physicians' handmaidens
rather than as independent practitioners. This perspective involves
more than just structural subordination; it casts the nurse in an assistant role rather than as a practitioner in her own right.

Incorporation, although potentially dangerous, does not have to
undermine the status of an occupation. American certified nurse-
midwives regard their additional training as a qualification for specialized, more highly skilled practice rather than merely the completion of prior nurse training. Their view parallels that of all medical
specialists who, while incorporated under the umbrella occupation of

medicine, see their specialties as distinct professions. For an incorporated occupation to retain its self-image as an independent specialty, it must provide intensive training to novices chosen on the basis of their career commitment to the field.

CAN INDEPENDENT MIDWIFERY SURVIVE LIMITATION TO THE NORMAL?

Unlike practitioners in other maternity care occupations when they emerged, modern independent midwives do not claim greater expertise in managing complications. Instead, they stress the inherent wellness of most pregnancies and the rarity of complications. Midwives claim knowledge of how to recognize incipient problems, not how to treat them. As a result, the maternity care that independent midwives offer combines passive monitoring of normal childbirth with time-consuming, individual emotional support, and with education about how nutrition, exercise, and rest can reduce the risk of complications.

Physicians often mistakenly assume that independent midwives represent a rebirth of the traditional midwives who flourished when health care was still largely a domestic function. This false impression stems from the out-of-hospital location of their work and their lack of claim to expertise in managing complications. Modern independent midwives make no such claim not, like traditional midwives, because they are ignorant of procedures but because they believe that experts already exist in more than ample number. They feel that this surplus of high risk experts has resulted in excessive, and sometimes dangerous, medicalization of births. Independent midwives practice in homes or free-standing clinics either because they have been excluded from practicing in hospitals or because they think it impossible to maintain a definition of childbirth as normal in the medically dominated hospital environment.

In reality the service offered by independent midwives is neither totally demedicalized nor a true alternative, as is chiropractic medicine. Instead, these midwives view maternity care as a continuum and want the legal right to serve women at the low risk end who want a natural childbirth. They do not reject the medical perspective that pathology can develop during pregnancy and childbirth. Nor do they have an alternative theory about the causes of pathology, other than a greater concern about the physical and psychological side effects of routinized obstetrical intervention. They do hold a different philosophy about what constitutes high quality care in the absence of pathology, however. As a result, they stress consumer education and consumer responsibility for minimizing the risk of complications. Yet the preventive behaviors they promote are the same ones physicians advocate.

The focus on well maternity care instead of all maternity care sets independent midwives apart from other occupations that have won limited professional status. Most of the other occupations—dentistry and podiatry, for example—provide a full continuum of service within their limited area of practice. While some provide services that traditionally have been shunned by more elite physicians, the most important factor in achieving limited autonomy has been their lack of dependence on medicine, according to Freidson (1970:69). Moreover, gender was not an obstacle for these predominantly male practitioners as it is for independent midwives.

In essence independent midwives are encroaching on maternity care from the rear flank. In contrast, perinatologists and all previous new maternity-care occupations found their openings at the advancing front line of obstetrical intervention. Whether the midwives' strategy can succeed is problematic for several reasons. Obstetricians clearly recognize the threat posed by independent midwives. Unlike perinatologists, who work from referrals, independent midwives compete directly with obstetricians for clients. Moreover, midwives' potential clientele is far larger than perinatologists' because considerably more pregnant women can be classified as low risk than high risk according to typical licensure standards. There also is far greater potential for a proliferation of independent midwives than perinatologists because of the considerably lower educational requirements and costs of training.

Obstetricians have responded to this threat by asserting their social and legal authority to determine the boundary between normal and abnormal childbirth. They have argued cogently that they are more qualified than midwives to determine the potential hazards of birth because they know more about the physiology of pathology. Although independent midwives feel that physicians generally diagnose abnormalities too quickly when any deviations from the norm occur and create complications by intervening unnecessarily, they lack authority on these issues because they claim no expertise about complications. Therefore their competitors define the boundaries of their work, leaving them highly vulnerable to economic pressures.

Their restriction to wellness care also makes independent midwives ultimately dependent on obstetricians' cooperation in providing assistance when problems arise. Even in the absence of legal subordination, midwives need sympathetic physicians to provide medical consultation and to treat their clients in hospitals when medical problems develop. And even where midwives have gained the legal right to work, their practices remain vulnerable to physicians' willingness to supply essential medical support.

CAN INDEPENDENT MIDWIFERY SURVIVE THE CHANGING CONTEXT OF HEALTH CARE?

In view of the problems inherent in claiming expertise only in normal childbirth, will history look back on the emergence of independent midwives as a false labor? For American midwives, the answer to this question depends on the changing context of health care delivery as well as the problem of defending the territory of an occupation based on wellness care.

The growth of independent midwifery derives from a broader disenchantment with modern health care. The last century has seen the proliferation of highly specialized physicians and the medicalization of many areas of life, including childbirth. At the same time chronic, degenerative disease and mental illness have replaced infectious disease as the major health problems in the Western world. The underlying behavioral and environmental components of these illnesses make them difficult to manage medically. Yet medical interventions—tonsillectomies, hysterectomies, mastectomies, coronary bypass surgeries, carotid artery strippings, and the prescription of tranquilizers and antidepressants, to name a few—achieved widespread adoption, some without proved therapeutic results. The cost of such treatments has led third-party payers to question physician authority. At the same time, a small but growing number of consumers have begun to seek new kinds of health care aimed at minimizing the risk of chronic disease, maximizing mental health, and assuming responsibility for their own physical health. Independent midwives may be the vanguard of a new group of wellness care practitioners evolving to serve this demand.

While social norms about health care are changing in a direction favorable to independent midwives, these practitioners may find their quest for a permanent share of maternity care undermined by changes in the organization of American health care (for a detailed discussion see: Starr, 1982:420–49). Public subsidy of medical costs for the elderly, poor, and disabled beginning in the mid-1960s made health care an attractive field for business investment. As a result, corporations began buying hospitals, nursing homes, and medical supply firms. The new corporate managers have a different perspective on health care delivery than the directors of traditional voluntary and public hospitals, who viewed their role as community service. Corporate managers instead view health care as a diversified product line that needs to be tailored to a splintered market of consumer preferences. To increase their competitive advantage and maximize their reimbursement, they have developed home health care services, life care retirement communities, specialty centers for services such as dialysis, and satellite ambulatory centers offering primary care in direct competition with private physicians. More recently they have ventured beyond acute care into prevention with behavioral modification programs for diet, smoking, substance abuse, and stress management. Some have merged with one another and with insurance companies to form huge, politically powerful conglomerates. They even have opened international operations in Britain, Australia, and other countries. Faced with such well-endowed competition benefiting from economies of scale, many nonprofit hospital groups have adopted similar expansionist strategies and acquired for-profit subsidiaries. If the process of corporatization continues, private practitioners, whether physicians or independent midwives, may be an endangered species because the high cost of equipment and malpractice insurance has made it increasingly difficult to compete against corporations.

Although the prospects for independent practice may be dimming, very recent changes in the financing of health may spell new opportunities for midwives as salaried employees. The continued escalation of fee-for-service charges in spite of declining inflation in the 1980s created a demand from a coalition of powerful groups—government, insurance carriers, and employers—for greater rationalization of health care services. The response has been a rapid growth in organizations which provide comprehensive health care for a prepaid fee and the introduction of set fees based on initial diagnosis rather than services rendered. These new financing arrangements combined with corporate interest in generating profit and funds for expansion are increasing the pressure to hold down provider costs while expanding utilization. Corporate managers have begun to respond by combining the marketing of new health care programs with policies to minimize hospitalization and medical intervention and maximize the use of paramedical personnel. Physicians who work as salaried employees are not in a position to stem the movement toward hiring paramedical workers, because corporations value their own financial needs over physicians' professional self-interest.

Corporations' willingness to use midwives is heightened by economic incentives to meet consumer demands. Many responded to the rise in midwife-attended home births by decorating some hospital rooms in a home-like style and aggressively advertising them as the best of both worlds—a home-like atmosphere safely located in the hospital. Some even hired certified nurse-midwives to staff the birthing rooms. Satellite free-standing birth centers would be a logical addition, as would postpartum home health services following the European model.

The history of midwifery in other Western developed countries suggests that the new employment opportunities arising from changes in the financing of American health care will be available only to nurse-midwives. If the wages are good and jobs plentiful and if the nurse-midwives are given some functional autonomy in the absence of complications, more lay midwives are likely to become certified nurse-midwives, further draining the ranks of independent practitioners.

The new financing arrangements should secure a place in maternity care for American midwives. But security may cost them much of their independence if their practices are constrained, like those of British midwives, by rigid treatment protocols. The bureaucratic environment also may cost them some of their alternative, holistic philosophy and individualized, passive management practices. As the experience of hospital birthing rooms has demonstrated, while the decor of home birth can be duplicated easily in institutional settings, the philosophy and practices cannot. Finally, should obstetrician-gynecologists succeed in becoming women's primary attendants and perinatologists take over obstetrics, salaried American midwives may follow their European counterparts and gradually devolve into nursing assistants.

If this happens, the rise of all modern midwifery, and not just independent midwifery, will indeed be a false labor.

REFERENCES

DeVries, Raymond G. *Regulating Birth: Midwives, Medicine and the Law.* Philadelphia: Temple University Press, 1985.

Foote, John. "Legislative measures against maternal and infant mortality: The midwife practice laws of the states and territories of the United States." *American Journal of Obstetrics and Diseases of Women and Children* 80:534–51, 1919.

Freidson, Elliot. *Profession of Medicine.* New York: Dodd, Mead, 1970.

Speert, Harold. *Obstetrics and Gynecology in America: A History.* Baltimore: Waverly Press, 1980.

Starr, Paul. *The Social Transformation of American Medicine.* New York: Basic Books, 1982.

White House Conference on Child Health and Protection. *Obstetric Education.* New York: The Century Co., 1932.

World Health Organization. *Having a Baby in Europe.* Public Health in Europe 26. Denmark, 1985.

INDEX

Accoucheurs. *See* Man-midwives; Obstetricians

American Academy of Pediatrics: pain relief medication, 31; pregnancy weight gain, 34; breastfeeding, 38; family-centered maternity care, 38; free-standing birth centers, 145

American College of Nurse-Midwives: relation to the American College of Obstetricians and Gynecologists, 18; family-centered care, 38. *See also* Certified nurse-midwives

American College of Obstetricians and Gynecologists: pain relief medication, 31; pregnancy weight gain, 34; family-centered maternity care, 38; home birth outcomes, 113, 133; statement on home birth, 142; hospital birth rooms, 143; free-standing birth centers, 145

American Medical Association: nineteenth-century view on obstetrics, 5; campaign against midwives, 9; opposition to Sheppard–Towner Maternity and Infancy Protection Act, 13

Amniocentesis, 37

Antibiotics, 25, 35, 174*n*

Antiseptic measures: nineteenth century, 8–9; mid-twentieth century, 25–26

Arizona School for Midwifery, 65

Arney, William, 168

Association of Radical Midwives, 177, 199

Barber-surgeons: and childbirth, 2–3, 4, 167, 202

Birth:
—attendants: twentieth century, 1, 14; colonial, 2–3; nineteenth century, 3–6
—centers: in hospitals, 143–44, 213, 214; free standing, 144–46, 204, 213
—location, change of, 1, 23
—publications, 68–69. *See also* Childbirth education; Natural childbirth; *specific childbirth groups*

Bonding, 30, 34, 38, 41, 162; research, 32–33; desire for, 36

Bottle feeding. *See* Infant formula

Breastfeeding: and antiseptic practices, 26; changing rates, 26; re-